Sirtfood Diet

This Book Includes:
Sirtfood Diet for Beginners and Cookbook.
The Complete Guide to Sirt Foods to Lose Weight and Burn Fat with Easy and Delicious Recipes and Weekly Meal Plans

Molly Ross

Text Copyright©

All rights reserved. No part of this guide may be reproduced in any form without permission in writing from the publisher except in the case of brief quotations embodied in critical articles or reviews.

Legal & Disclaimer

The information contained in this book and its contents is not designed to replace or take the place of any form of medical or professional advice; and is not meant to replace the need for independent medical, financial, legal or other professional advice or services, as may be required. The content and information in this book has been provided for educational and entertainment purposes only.

The content and information contained in this book has been compiled from sources deemed reliable, and it is accurate to the best of the Author's knowledge, information and belief. However, the Author cannot guarantee its accuracy and validity and cannot be held liable for any errors and/or omissions. Further, changes are periodically made to this book as and when needed. Where appropriate and/or necessary, you must consult a professional (including but not limited to your doctor, attorney, financial advisor or such other professional advisor) before using any of the suggested remedies, techniques, or information in this book.

Upon using the contents and information contained in this book, you agree to hold harmless the Author from and against any damages, costs, and expenses, including any legal fees potentially resulting from the application of any of the information provided by this book. This disclaimer applies to any loss, damages or injury caused by the use and application, whether directly or indirectly, of any advice or information presented, whether for breach of contract, tort, negligence, personal injury, criminal intent, or under any other cause of action.

You agree to accept all risks of using the information presented inside this book.

You agree that by continuing to read this book, where appropriate and/or necessary, you shall consult a professional (including but not limited to your doctor, attorney, or financial advisor or such needed) before using any of the suggested remedies, techniques, or information in this book.

Table of Contents: Sirtfood Diet for Beginners

Introduction 13

Chapter 1: Sirtfoods And Sirtuins 23

Chapter 2: How to Build A Diet That Works 30

Chapter 3: Top Sirtfoods 36

Chapter 4: Benefits of Sirtfoods 44

Chapter 5: Sirtfood Diet – Phase 1 53

Chapter 6: Sirtfood Diet – Phase 2 63

Chapter 7: Sirtfood For Life - Sustainability and Benefits 73

Chapter 8: Questions and Answers 83

Chapter 9: Sirtfood Recipes 88

Conclusion 129

Table of Contents: Sirtfood Diet Cookbook

Introduction	**135**
The Sirtfood Diet	**138**
1. Fun Facts about Sirtuins	139
2. The Discovery and History of Sirtuins	141
Benefits of Sirtfoods	**144**
3. Top 20 Sirtfoods	144
4. Appetite for Fasting	145
5. An Energy for Exercise	146
Sirtfood Diet– Phase 1 & Phase 2	**149**
6. Phase 1 (The Most Effective): Three Kilos in Seven Days	149
7. Phase 2 (Maintenance), For 14 Days	150
Breakfast Recipes – Phase 1	**154**
1. Main Baby Spinach Snack	154
2. Potato Bites	155
3. Sesame Dip	156
4. Rosemary Squash Dip	157
5. Bean Spread	158
6. Eggplant Salsa	159
7. Carrots and Cauliflower Spread	160
8. Italian Veggie Salsa	161
9. Black Bean Salsa	162
10. Corn Spread	163
11. Mushroom Dip	164
12. Salsa Bean Dip	165
13. Mung Sprouts Salsa	166
14. Mung Beans Snack Salad	167
15. Sprouts and Apples Snack Salad	168
Main Meals Recipes – Phase 1	**170**
16. Salmon and Capers	170

17. Coconut curry — 171
18. Tofu Thai Curry — 172
19. Turkey Curry — 174
20. Sirtfood Pizza — 175
21. Red Coleslaw — 177
22. Avocado Mayo Medley — 178
23. Amazing Garlic Aioli — 179
24. Easy Seed Crackers — 180

Main Meals Recipes – Phase 1 (Part 2) — 183
25. Sticky Chicken Watermelon Noodle Salad — 183
26. Fruity Curry Chicken Salad — 186
27. Zuppa Toscana — 187
28. Turmeric Chicken & Kale Salad with Honey-Lime Dressing — 189
29. Buckwheat Noodles with Chicken Kale — 192
30. Asian King Prawn with Buckwheat Noodles — 194

Dessert Recipes – Phase 1 — 197
31. Creamy Strawberry & Cherry Smoothie — 197
32. Grape, Celery & Parsley Reviver — 198
33. Strawberry & Citrus Blend — 199
34. Chocolate Hazelnut Brownie Pie — 200
35. Slice-and-Bake Vanilla Wafers — 201
36. Amaretti — 202
37. Peanut Butter Cookies for Two — 203
38. Cream Cheese Cookies — 204
39. Chewy Double Chocolate Cookies — 205
40. Mocha Cream Pie — 206
41. Coconut Custard Pie — 207
42. Dairy-Free Fruit Tarts — 208

Other Recipes – Phase1 — 210
43. Apple & Celery Juice — 210
44. Broccoli, Apple, & Orange Juice — 211
45. Green Fruit Juice — 212

46. Kale & Fruit Juice	213
47. Kale, Carrot, & Grapefruit Juice	214
48. Buckwheat Granola	215
49. Apple Pancakes	217
50. Matcha Pancakes	219
51. Smoked Salmon & Kale Scramble	221
52. Kale & Mushroom Frittata	222
53. Kale, Apple, & Cranberry Salad	224
54. Arugula, Strawberry, & Orange Salad	225
55. Beef & Kale Salad	226
Breakfast Recipes – Phase 2	**229**
56. Green Omelette	229
57. Berry Oat Breakfast Cobbler	230
58. Pancakes with Apples and Blackcurrants	231
59. Granola- The Sirt Way	233
60. Summer Berry Smoothie	234
61. Mango, Celery & Ginger Smoothie	235
62. Orange, Carrot & Kale Smoothie	236
63. Creamy Strawberry & Cherry Smoothie	237
64. Grape, Celery & Parsley Reviver	238
65. Strawberry & Citrus Blend	239
66. Grapefruit & Celery Blast	240
67. Orange & Celery Crush	241
68. Tropical Chocolate Delight	242
69. Walnut & Spiced Apple Tonic	243
70. Pineapple & Cucumber Smoothie	244
Main Meals Recipes – Phase 2	**246**
71. Honey Chili Squash	246
72. Chicken & Bean Casserole	247
73. Roast Balsamic Vegetables	248
74. Mussels in Red Wine Sauce	249
Main Meals Recipes – Phase 2 (Part 2)	**251**

75. Courgette Risotto	251
76. Chilli Con Carne	252
77. Brown Basmati Rice Pilaf	255
78. Thai Red Curry	256
79. Artichoke & Eggplant Rice	258
Dessert Recipes – Phase 2	**261**
80. Apple-Raisin Cake	261
81. Apple-Nut Squares	263
82. Yogurt-Fruit Pie	265
83. Potato Rosettes	267
84. Creamy Peanut Dip	268
85. Stuffed Dates	269
Other Recipes – Phase 1	**271**
86. Soup 'Green	271
87. Pea Salad, Gourmet Peas, Grapefruit	273
88. Detoxifying Milkshake	275
89. Green Pineapple Smoothie	276
90. Cream of Pear and Arugula	277
91. Chocolate Cupcakes with Matcha Icing-Sirt Food	279
Other Recipes – Phase 1 (Part 2)	**282**
92. Creamy Strawberry & Cherry Smoothie	282
93. Grapefruit & Celery Blast	283
94. Orange & Celery Crush	284
95. Tropical Chocolate Delight	285
96. Walnut & Spiced Apple Tonic	286
97. Coq Au Vin	287
98. Turkey Satay Skewers	288
99. Salmon & Capers	289
100. Moroccan Chicken Casserole	290
101. Chili Con Carne	291
102. Prawn & Coconut Curry	292
103. Choc Nut Truffles	293

104. No-Bake Strawberry Flapjacks	294
105. Chocolate Balls	295
Two-Week Meal Plan – Phase 1 and Phase 2	**297**
Phase 1	297
Day 1-3	297
Day 1: Monday	297
Day 2: Tuesday	297
Day 3: Wednesday	298
Day 4–7	298
Day 4: Thursday	298
Day 5: Friday	298
Day 6: Saturday	299
Day 7: Sunday	299
Phase 2	299
Day 8 and 15	300
Day 9 and 16	300
Day 10 and 17	301
Day 11 and 18	301
Day 12 and 19	302
Day 13 and 20	302
Day 14 and 21	303
Conclusion	**305**

Sirtfood Diet for Beginners

The Complete Guide to Sirt Foods to Activate Your Skinny Gene, Lose Weight Fast, and Burn Fat with Easy and Delicious Recipes for Your Meal Plan

Molly Ross

Introduction

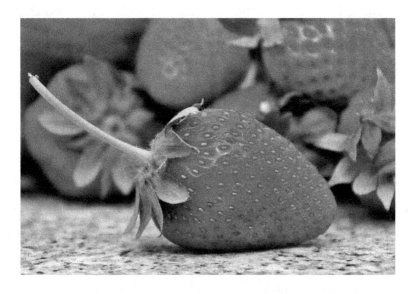

Sirtuins are a type of protein that safeguards the cells in our bodies from dying or becoming swollen through disease, though research study has actually likewise shown they can help control your metabolism, increase muscle, and burn fat-- hence the new 'wonder-food' tag. Sirtfoods is a recently identified group of foods that have an effective recycling process in the body that clears cellular waste and burns fat. Together with fat-burning, Sirtfoods likewise have the distinct capability to naturally satisfy hunger and boost muscle function, making them the ideal service to accomplishing a healthy weight. And their health improving impacts are so effective that research studies reveal them to be more powerful than prescription drugs in preventing chronic illness, with benefits in diabetes, heart problem and Alzheimer's to simply call a few. It is no marvel that it is well developed that the cultures consuming the most Sirtfoods have been the cleanest and healthiest on the planet.

In the last few years, fasting diets have actually been the most significant fad, notable ones like the 5:2 diet plan, which was the-diet-to-do in 2015.

But the Sirtfood plan is expected to mimic the weight-loss results of a fasting diet plan-- but without jeopardizing health, physical fitness, and muscle mass or food fulfillment, thanks to brand-new research into this food group. Just in case 500-calorie Mondays (AKA hungry-all-day Mondays) did not actually work out for you. Although being an efficient weight loss program, the writers are eager to stress that it is not just a diet plan, however a wellbeing and fitness regime.

"It doesn't need calorie limitation, nor does it demand grueling exercise programs (although obviously, usually staying active is a good idea). It's neither pricey nor lengthy, and all the foods we suggest are widely readily available."

And yes, in that list consists of dark chocolate (cocoa) and red, white wine - rejoice!

Introduction

It is the buzz diet plan of 2016, and already a preferred amongst celebrities, with everybody from Jodie Kidd to Lorraine Pascal liking it.

Lorraine named it "a non-faddy diet plan that offers extraordinary health benefits and weight-loss."

Jodie stated: "Since following it, I feel unstoppable."

How exactly do these foods work to attain such outcomes?

Sirtuin

Sirtuins help manage the health of your cell phones. This is what you need to know about how you work, what you can do for your body, and why you depend on NAD+ to work.

Sirtuins are a class of cell safety proteins. Sirtuins may work only with NAD+, a coenzyme found in all living cells, nicotinamide adenine dinucleotide.

How Sirtuins Regulate Cellular Health with NAD+.

Think about your body's cells like a workplace. In the office, there are lots of people dealing with various jobs with the ultimate goal: remain lucrative and satisfy the objective of the business in an effective way for as long as possible. In the cells, several workpieces operate on various activities with an ultimate goal as well: they remain healthy and perform as long as possible effectively.

Essentially as the top priorities of progress in the organization are issues in the cells, because of various internal and external factors.

Someone must manage the office, control what happens where who will and when to travel. That would be your CEO in the office. In the body, it is your sirtuins at the cellular level.

Sirtuins are a class of seven proteins that have a cell health role.

NAD+ is crucial to cellular metabolic process and numerous other biological procedures. If the sirtuins are the CEO of a firm, then NAD+ is the cash spent by the CEO and staff while keeping the lights on and having the office rent paid. A company, and the body, cannot operate without it. Levels of NAD+ decrease with age, restricting the function of sirtuins with age. Like all things in the body, it is not that basic. Sirtuins handle everything that occurs in your cells.

Sirtuins Are Proteins. What Does That Mean?

Sirtuins are a household of proteins. Protein might sound like dietary protein-- what is found in meats and beans, and well, protein shakes-- however, in this case we are discussing molecules called proteins, which work throughout the body's cells in a variety of various functions. Think about proteins as the departments at a business, each one concentrating on its own particular function while coordinating with other departments.

A widely known protein in the body is hemoglobin, which belongs to the globin family of proteins and is responsible for transferring oxygen throughout your blood. Myoglobin is the equivalent of the hemoglobin, and together they comprise the global household.

Introduction

Your body has almost 60,000 families of proteins-- a great deal of departments! -- and sirtuins are among those families. While hemoglobin is one in a household of 2 proteins, sirtuins are a household of seven.

Myoglobin is the equivalent of the hemoglobin, and together they comprise the global household.

Acetyl groups control specific responses. These are actual marks of proteins that are recognized by other proteins. While proteins are cell divisions and DNA are Chairman, the acetyl groups are each department head's schedule position. For example, if a protein is readily available, then the sirtuin can work with it to make something happen, simply as the CEO can work with an offered department head to make something occur.

Sirtuins use deacetylation to work with acetyl groups. This means that they know that there is an acetyl group on a molecule and then remove the acetyl group which loads the molecule for its function. One-way sirtuins function is to get rid of biological proteins such as histones in acetyl groups (deacetylating). Make it a Christmas tree and the fur of the lights is the DNA line. If the histones have a community of acetyls, chromatin is free or unwound.

This unwound chromatin implies the process of transcription of the DNA. It does not have to remain unwound because it is prone to damages, almost like Christmas lights, or when they are unmanageable or up for too long, bulbs can be destroyed. When the histones are deacetylated by sirtuins, the chromatin is blocked, or the gene expression with sense is halted or silenced firmly and beautifully.

We have just understood about sirtuins for about 20 years, and their primary function was discovered in the 1990s. Because then, researchers have actually flocked to study them, identifying their value while likewise raising concerns about what else we can discover them.

The Discovery and History of Sirtuins
Geneticist Dr. Amar Klar found the first sirtuin, called SIR2, in the 1970s, identifying it as a gene that controlled the capability of yeast cells to mate. Years later, in the 1990s, scientists found other genes identical-similar in structure-to SIR2, which were then called sirtuins in other species such as worms and fruit flies. Each organism had different types of sirtuins. For eg, yeast has 5 sirtuins, one bacterium, seven mice and seven humans.

The fact that sirtuins were present in all habitats indicates that they have been "conserved." "Conserved" genes have similar roles in many or all forms. Nevertheless, what still needed to be known was how important sirtuins were to be.

In 1991, Leonard Guarantee, Elysium co-founder and MIT scientist, and Nick Austriaco and Brian Kennedy, graduate trainees, conducted experiments to learn how yeast aged more efficiently. By mistake, Austriaco was trying to develop colonies under various yeast strains from experiments that he had actually saved for months in his fridge, which created a complicated tension setting.

The strains of yeast that endured the very best in the refrigerator were also the longest-lived. This aided with Guarente so he might focus entirely on these long-living strains of yeast.

It is important to remember that up to now, there is no proof that this analysis can be extrapolated to humans and further work on the effect of SIR2 on humans is required. Consequently, the Guarente lab observed that the deletion of SIR2 substantially reduced the yeast life, while the number of copies of the SIR2 gene expanded by one to two, the yeast life span.

This is where acetyl groups enter play. It was at first thought that SIR2 might be a deacetylation enzyme-- indicating it eliminated those acetyl groups-- from other particles, but nobody knew if this were true considering that all attempts to show this activity in a test tube showed negative. Guarantee and his team found that SIR2 could actually deacetylate certain proteins in the life of the ND+ coenzyme nicotinamide adenine dinucleotide in yeast.

Guarente's own words: "SIR2 doesn't do anything without NAD+. That's the key finding in the arc of sirtuin biology."

The Future of Sirtuins
As the sirtuins field continues to broaden, this leaves space for amazing research study chances into how triggering sirtuins with NAD+ precursors can lead to more amazing discoveries.

Jadis Tillery was stressed over her waist in the run-up to her wedding last March. 'I have diabetes in my household, so I've constantly known the need to stay trim,' discusses the 32-year-old marketing executive from London.

' But despite the fact that I consume well and work out routinely, I just could not move those few extra pounds around my middle. Precisely the location my gown was going to highlight.'

She discovered a unique brand-new weekly diet plan - which included cutting her calories to simply 1,000 a day for 3 days, then increasing them to 1,500 for the remaining 4. (The normal suggested daily intake for a woman is 2,000).

The results, she states, were 'fantastic.' Not just did she hardly ever suffer cravings pangs (' For the last four days I was consuming 1,500 calories and having 2 scrumptious meals a day, but by the end of the week I was discovering it tough to finish them']; however, she had loads more energy.

A lot more pleasing was the physical results.

I understand about diet plans - I've been on plenty - but the outcomes came as a genuine surprise. By the end of the week, I 'd lost just over 6lb of fat. But the genuine shock was discovering that I 'd put on almost 2lb of muscle, although I 'd done essentially no workout because of time.'

This indicated her total weight reduction on the scales was 4lb, but her body structure had actually altered, so she was leaner. (This was computed by measuring her body fat with calipers prior to and after and then comparing that with the weight lost).

This is not the kind of outcome you should predict alone (and even then, you would not expect such a weight loss). So, what is going to happen?

The secret lies in what Jadis ate.

Her diet was full of naturally available foods in chemical compounds, which experts think are important for fat burning, cravings elimination, and health enhancement.

Chapter 1: Sirtfoods And Sirtuins

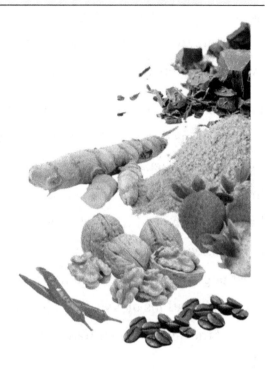

Sirtuins manage a wide scope of procedures, including interpretation, digestion, fat assembly, neurodegeneration and maturing. The different elements of these proteins have been to a great extent attributed to their capacity to catalyze the expulsion of acetyl bunches from the lysine amino-corrosive deposits of different proteins through their deacetylase movement. However, the definite natural activity of sirtuins stays vague. For example, one sirtuin, SIRT6, which has been ensnared in genome strength, irritation, malignant growth cell digestion and even lifespan, is an extremely powerless deacetylase1. On page 110 of this issue, Jiang et al.2 report the astounding revelation that SIRT6 heartily evacuates a myristoyl gathering — a long-chain greasy acyl gathering — from lysine deposits, and that this biochemical action empowers the chemical to manage the emission of TNF-α, a cytokine protein discharged from cells during irritation.

Proteins experience and assorted cluster of compound modifications that adjust their movement. The catalysts that include and evacuate these modifications are therefore key chiefs in flagging falls. The lysine side chains of proteins can be modified by connection of a little acyl bunch called acetyl, which is one of the most widely recognized administrative modifications and is most popular for its job in controlling interpretation. Other, bigger acyl modifications of lysine buildups have been distinguished, in spite of the fact that their natural jobs are to a great extent obscure.

The greater part of the seven human sirtuins (SIRT1–7) show this run of the mill movement, albeit a few, including SIRT6, have either powerless or no deacetylase action. For example, SIRT5 specially ties to and expels succinyl and malonyl modifications from lysine3. These acyl bunches are bigger than acetyls and, in contrast to them, are adversely charged, yet they are connected to lysine by a similar sort of compound bond and are evacuated in the equivalent NAD+-subordinate enzymatic response as that catalyzed by different sirtuins.

Sirtuins are referred to go about as deacetylase proteins. They evacuate the acyl gathering (R) acetyl from the lysine side chain of substrate proteins in a response including the NAD+ cofactor and move it to the rest of the ADP-ribose moiety of NAD+ (green) to frame O-acetyl ADP-ribose. (Nicotinamide is a side-effect of the response.) Jiang et al.2 report that SIRT6 specially evacuates a different, long-chain acyl gathering (myristoyl) from proteins — a finding that, together with past information, require a reclassification of sirtuins as deacylases.

The SIRT5 point of reference incited Jiang et al. to research whether the obviously powerless deacetylase action of SIRT6 likewise mirrors an inclination for other acyl-lysine substrates. Their pursuit started in vitro with the utilization of synthetically blended peptides bearing lysine modified with different acyl bunches that are known to happen in cells. The outcome was clear: SIRT6 was undeniably increasingly dynamic in evacuating the long-chain greasy acyl myristoyl and palmitoyl bunches than little acyl modifications, including acetyl gatherings.

The creators' precious stone structure of SIRT6 bound to a myristoylated peptide and ADP-ribose shows that SIRT6 contains an extended hydrophobic divert in which it can suit the 14-carbon myristoyl chain. Together with past basic studies3,4,5 indicating how different sirtuins can suit different acyl modifications, including succinyl, malonyl and propionyl lysine, it presently appears to be certain that auxiliary highlights in the sirtuins' dynamic locales oversee the inclination of everyone for expelling a specific kind of acyl modification.

In vivo, SIRT6 is known to direct the degrees of TNF-α, which traverses the cell film and is cut by a layer related protease compound, bringing about the emission of this current cytokine's extracellular area. The cytoplasmic area of TNF-α contains two myristoylated lysine. This quickly brings up two issues: does SIRT6 expel these myristoyl modifications and, if things being what they are, is this enzymatic action by one way or another associated with TNF-α guideline?

Without a doubt, Jiang et al. discovered that the myristylation level of TNF-α in refined cells relied upon the enzymatic movement of SIRT6. Emission of TNF-α likewise required SIRT6, demonstrating that expulsion of its myristoyl bunches is a key advance in this procedure. It will be intriguing to perceive how myristylation manages emission, and whether expulsion of the myristoyl bunches causes a conformational revamp in TNF-α that permits its cleavage by the layer related protease.

Jiang and associates' discoveries set up for a few new headings wherein to explore the job of greasy acyl modifications and their guideline by sirtuins. The paper ought to be the last driving force for reclassifying sirtuins as lysine deacylases5, and not just deacetylases, to mirror the broader nature of their enzymatic movement.

Significantly, it presently appears that sirtuins differ from each other in the kind of acyl modification they specially expel from substrates, albeit current discoveries do not decide out the likelihood that a given sirtuin can evacuate a few sorts of acyl modification in vivo. This is maybe the situation for SIRT6. In spite of the fact that the compound specially expels long-chain greasy acyl modifications, its deacetylase movement has been implicated6 in modification of the DNA-related histone H3 protein. It may be the case that, in vivo, the feeble deacetylase action of SIRT6 is confined to specific substrates (as has been shown6), to exact subcellular restrictions or to specific flagging pathways. The way that SIRT6 can expel a more extensive range of acyl modifications should make it conceivable to coax out the overall commitments of these biochemical exercises to this current chemical's capacity.

It has for quite some time been a riddle why sirtuins expend the vivaciously exorbitant NAD+ cofactor, as opposed to — like different classes of deacetylase — utilizing basic hydrolysis to deacetylate substrates. Clarifications summoned incorporate the administrative ramifications of coupling sirtuin movement to the phone's metabolic state, in which NAD+ is included, or the conceivable flagging job of the O-acetyl ADP-ribose item (Fig. 1). Another clarification might be the need to create a nucleotide bearer for the leaving acyl gathering. On moving from the lysine substrate to ADP-ribose to frame O-myristoyl ADP-ribose, the hydrophobic myristate is discharged in an increasingly solvent conjugated structure. The O-myristoyl ADP-ribose conjugation additionally forestalls myristate from getting lengthened by further enzymatic response to frame another unsaturated fat, palmitate, along these lines safeguarding the accessible pool of myristate.

O-Acetyl ADP-ribose is separated by a few enzymes7, and it is not yet clear which of them control the degrees of other O-acyl ADP-ribose items or move them to different bearers, and whether these exercises influence or even drive upstream pathways engaged with creating these metabolites. Until further notice, the disclosure of SIRT6-interceded demyristoylation opens an energizing section in the account of the seven human sirtuins and their natural action."

How to Build a diet that works

Chapter 2: How to Build A Diet That Works

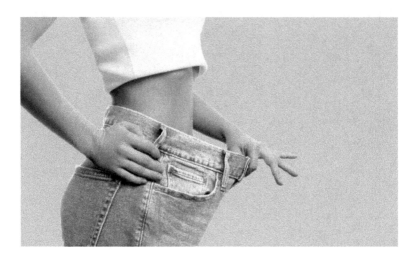

The basis of the sirtuin diet can be explained in simple terms or in complex ways. It is important to understand how and why it works however, so that you can appreciate the value of what you are doing. It is important to also know why these sirtuin rich foods help to help you maintain fidelity to your diet plan. Otherwise, you may throw something in your meal with less nutrition that would defeat the purpose of planning for one rich in sirtuins. Most importantly, this is not a dietary fad, and as you will see, there is much wisdom contained in how humans have used natural foods even for medicinal purposes, over thousands of years.

To understand how the Sirtfood diet works, and why these particular foods are necessary, we will look at the role they play in the human body.

Sirtuin activity was first researched in yeast, where a mutation caused an extension in the yeast's lifespan. Sirtuins were also shown to slow aging in laboratory mice, fruit flies, and nematodes. As research on Sirtuins proved to transfer to mammals, they were examined for their use in diet and slowing the aging process. The sirtuins in humans are different in the typing but they essentially work in the same ways and reasons.

There are seven "members" that make up the sirtuin family. It is believed that sirtuins play a big role in regulating certain functions of cells including proliferation (reproduction and growth of cells), apoptosis (death of cells). They promote survival and resist stress to increase longevity.

They are also seen to block neurodegeneration (loss or function of the nerve cells in the brain). They conduct their housekeeping functions by cleaning out toxic proteins and supporting the brain's ability to change and adapt to different conditions, or to recuperate (i.e., brain plasticity). As part of this they also help reduce chronic inflammation and reduce something called oxidative stress. Oxidative stress is when there are too many cell-damaging free radicals circulating in the body, and the body cannot catch up by combating them with antioxidants. These factors are related to age-related illness and weight as well, which again, brings us back to a discussion of how they actually work.

You will see labels in Sirtuins that start with "SIR," which represents "Silence Information Regulator" genes. They do exactly that, silence or regulate, as part of their functions. The seven sirtuins that humans work with are: SIRT1, SIRT2, SIRT3, SIRT4, SIRT 5, SIRT6 and SIRT7. Each of these types is responsible for different areas of protecting cells. They work by either stimulating or turning on certain gene expressions, or by reducing and turning off other gene expressions. This essentially means that they can influence genes to do more or less of something, most of which they are already programmed to do.

Through enzyme reactions, each of the SIRT types affects different areas of cells that are responsible for the metabolic processes that help to maintain life. This is also related to what organs and functions they will affect.

For example, the SIRT6 causes an expression of genes in humans that affect skeletal muscle, fat tissue, brain, and heart. SIRT 3 would cause an expression of genes that affect the kidneys, liver, brain, and heart.

If we tie these concepts together, you can see that the Sirtuin proteins can change the expression of genes, and in the case of the Sirtfood diet we care about how sirtuins can turn off those genes that are responsible for speeding up aging and for weight management.

The other aspect to this conversation of sirtuins is the function and the power of calorie restriction on the human body. Calorie restriction is simply eating fewer calories. This coupled with exercise and reducing stress is usually a combination for weight loss. Calorie restriction has also proven across much research in animals and humans to increase one's lifespan.

We can look further at the role of sirtuins with calorie restriction and using the SIRT3 protein which has a role in metabolism and aging.

The SIRT3 has high expression in those metabolically active tissues as we stated earlier, and its ability to express itself increases with caloric restriction, fasting, and exercise. On the contrary, it will express itself less when the body has a high fat, high calorie-riddled diet.

The last few highlights of sirtuins are their role in regulating telomeres and reducing inflammation which also help with staving off disease and aging.

Telomeres are sequences of proteins at the ends of chromosomes. When cells divide these get shorter. As we age, they get shorter and other stressors to the body also will contribute to this. Maintaining these longer telomeres is the key to slower aging. In addition, proper diet, along with exercise and other variables can lengthen telomeres. SIRT6 is one of the sirtuins that, if activated, can help with DNA damage, inflammation, and oxidative stress.

SIRT1 also helps with inflammatory response cycles that are related to many age-related diseases.

Calories restriction, as we mentioned earlier, can extend life to some degree.

Since this, as well as fasting, is a stressor, these factors will stimulate the SIRT3 proteins to kick in and protect the body from the stressors and excess free radicals. Again, the telomere length is affected as well.

To sum up, all of this information also shows that, contrary to some people's beliefs that in terms of genetics, such as "it is what it is" or "it is my fate because Uncle Joe has something…" through our own lifestyle choices, and what we are exposed to, we can influence action and changes in our genes. This is quite an empowering thought, and yet another reason why you should be excited to have a science-based diet such as the Sirtfood diet, available to you.

How to Build a diet that works

Chapter 3: Top Sirtfoods

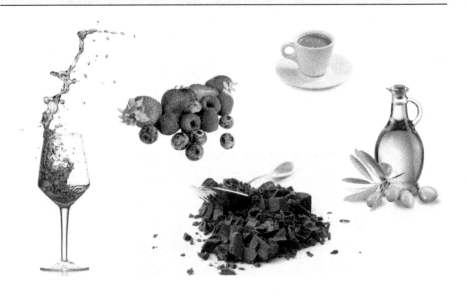

As of late, you may have known about the Sirtfood Diet, the popular eating regimen that guarantees you can lose as much as 7 pounds in 7 days. Established by U.K. sustenance specialists Aidan Goggins and Glen Matten, the Sirtfood Diet vows to invigorate the "thin quality," or the proteins under the SIRT1 quality, to check the impacts of aggravation and weight gain, just as maturing.

The Sirtfood Diet depends on the rule that specific nourishments enact sirtuin, a (profoundly questionable) protein in the body that is claimed to help control digestion and offer cell security to hinder the maturing procedure.

The Sirtfood Diet is part into two stages. The main stage, which keeps going three days, expects you to confine your day by day calorie admission to 1000 calories for every day by drinking three green juices and one sirtfood-rich feast every day. (You increment your dinner check from days 4 to 7 to two suppers and two green juices for every day.) The subsequent stage, the "support" stage, keeps going 14 days and expects you to eat three sirtuin-rich dinners and one green juice for every day.

While the guarantee of the Sirtfood diet is interesting (Adele and Pippa Middleton are apparently fans), and keeping in mind that confining your calories may in reality lead you to shed pounds for the time being, the inquiry remains: is this eating regimen really solid, or is it simply one more senseless (and conceivably hazardous) diet pattern? So far as that is concerned, is it even successful in any case?

First: the Sirtfood diet is as a matter of fact exceptionally prohibitive. In contrast to the Keto or Paleo consumes less calories, which underscore having a decent eating regimen, the Sirtfood diet centers vigorously around tallying calories. It additionally expects you to remove some significant nutritional categories and scale back bits to an extraordinary, if just incidentally. So, for the main week or something like that, you may be passing up lean proteins (hamburger, poultry, and vegetables). While you're despite everything permitted to eat olive oil and pecan (the two of which are wellsprings of sirtuin), the complete day by day carbohydrate content for the main week is incredibly low — under half of what the normal dynamic person needs. It additionally needs other fundamental supplements, like calcium and iron.

It is likewise vague whether sirtuin can really cause weight reduction regardless. Until this point in time, there have been no human investigations absolutely connecting sirtuin-rich nourishments to weight reduction. All things considered, drinking juices that are high in greens and low in sugar for a large portion of the day can without much of a stretch reason transient weight reduction all alone: in case you're getting less calories and remaining hydrated, it bodes well that you'll shed a couple of pounds.

Kristen Smith, MS, RD, LD, a representative for the Academy of Nutrition and Dietetics, backs this up. "It is hard to unravel whether the quick weight reduction guaranteed in the primary seven day stretch of the eating routine is ascribed to the altogether low-calorie diet prescribed or identified with the fat-consuming forces of sirtuin-boosting nourishments," she says.

Fundamentally, "paying little heed to the sirtuin-boosting nourishments, individuals will shed pounds on a 1000-calorie diet," she clarifies.

Alpert concurs. "The creators state that individuals can lose as much as 7 pounds in 7 days, yet I wonder the amount of this weight really remains off for longer than one month, if that long," she clarifies.

Regardless of whether you get in shape during that first week, it could be essentially water weight, which implies you may recover it once you begin taking in more calories. Truth be told, you may even put on more weight: as Men's Health has recently announced, when you lose a great deal of weight rapidly, your body's digestion really eases back down, on the grounds that your body is attempting to compensate for its decreased calorie consumption.

Likewise, with any eating regimen, the Sirtfood Diet additionally accompanies its own reactions. While it likely won't do a lot of harm for you to eat so little for the time being, in case you're not used to eating so small during the day, it can cause exhaustion, sickness, weakened mental center, and cerebral pains, says Smith. It can likewise prompt horrendous defecations in case you are not getting enough fiber. Likewise, you may get terrible breath, which can be a reaction of not eating enough.

There is, in any case, one positive: If you eat a great deal of sirtfoods over a continued timeframe, you may see enhancements in heart wellbeing due to the polyphenols in the nourishments you are eating, Smith says. If you keep on eating sirtfoods after you end the eating routine and begin to eat more calories, you will see the advantages.

The takeaway? While it is probably going to prompt transient weight reduction, the Sirtfood diet is eventually so prohibitive that it is not so much reasonable. Also, if you've at any point had a dietary issue or a confounded association with eating previously, it is ideal to keep away from it out and out, says Alpert.

"I wouldn't prescribe such a low-calorie admission for anybody. Extraordinary eating less junk food sets individuals up for horrible dietary patterns and indulging when it's finished," she includes.

All things considered, eating more sirtuin-rich nourishments is without a doubt useful for your wellbeing, so you can undoubtedly bring them into your eating regimen without restricting yourself to each dinner or one squeeze in turn. There's nothing amiss with eating more fish, berries, and verdant greens (particularly in light of the fact that these nourishments are stuffed with fiber and protein) and having a green squeeze that is low in sugar could be an incredible expansion to a previously adjusted eating routine.

At last, you can presumably receive the rewards of the SIRT diet without making a plunge totally. Simply ensure your bits are reasonable and you are getting your calories from a wide assortment of solid sources — no accident eating less junk food or juice fasting important.

The Sirtfood diet has produced a tremendous buzz, just as a top spot on the Amazon smash hit diagrams. With claims that 'sirtfoods' (of which cocoa and red wine are incorporated) "switch on your muscle versus fat's consuming forces, supercharge weight reduction and assist fight with offing ailment", and that the eating regimen could assist you with losing 7lbs in seven days, it's no big surprise individuals are paying heed.

In any case, for the more distrustful among us, it is enticing to hold this eating routine alongside the large number of other "prevailing fashion" weight reduction designs that have gone before it.

Be that as it may, the sirtfood diet professes to be established in science, with more than 100 referenced investigations to back it up, which has made skeptical specialists sit up and give more consideration. So, what precisely are these sirtfoods, and how would they work (if at all...)?

These "thin qualities" are known as sirtuins, a class of proteins that examination has demonstrated to be significant for managing natural pathways which influence our wellbeing and weight.

The writers proceed to depict how "sirtfoods go about as ace controllers of our digestion, most having impacts on fat consuming while at the same time expanding muscle and improving cell wellness."

The best 20 sirtfoods are:

1. Additional virgin olive oil
2. Tricks
3. Red onions
4. Parsley
5. Kale
6. Pecans
7. Strawberries
8. Bean stew
9. Soy items
10. Cocoa
11. Green tea
12. Espresso
13. Medjool dates
14. Red chicory
15. lovage
16. Rocket
17. Celery
18. Buckwheat
19. Turmeric
20. Red wine

Benefits of Sirtfoods

Chapter 4: Benefits of Sirtfoods

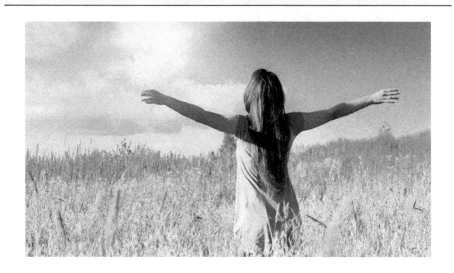

What are the advantages?

You will get more fit on the off chance that you follow this eating regimen intently. "Regardless of whether you're eating 1,000 calories of tacos, 1,000 calories of kale, or 1,000 calories of snickerdoodles, you will get more fit at 1,000 calories!" says Dr Youdim. In any case, she additionally brings up that you can have accomplishment with a progressively sensible calorie limitation. The run of the mill every day caloric admission of somebody not on an eating routine is 2,000 to 2,200, so decreasing to 1,500 is as yet confining and would be a successful weight reduction procedure for most, she says.

Are there any safety measures?

This arrangement is severe with little squirm room or substitutions, and weight reduction must be kept up if the low caloric admission is likewise kept up, making it hard to hold fast to the long haul. That implies any weight you lost in the initial seven days is probably going to be recovered after you finish, says Dr Youdin. Her primary concern? "Constraining protein admission with juices will bring about lost bulk. Losing muscle is synonymous with dropping your metabolic rate or 'digestion,' making weight upkeep increasingly troublesome," she says.

What do practical nourishment specialists need to state about it?

Generally speaking, master input on the Sirtfood Diet is blended. The uplifting news: The eating regimen seems to be stacked with sound nourishments. "There is broad research that features the numerous advantages of a portion of the nourishments got down on about this eating routine, similar to espresso, green tea, dull chocolate, and dim verdant greens," says Jessica Cording, R.D., enrolled dietitian and wellbeing mentor.

Vast numbers of these nourishments may likewise bolster substantial weight reduction, says Frances Large man-Roth, R.D., however, whether they advance weight reduction by actuating sirtuins stays to be demonstrated. "The nourishments advanced on the eating routine are ones that battle aggravation and would be valuable for anybody to add to their eating regimen yet not because they help sirtuins," she says. "Because nourishment contains a specific supplement connected to digestion doesn't imply that nourishment causes programmed weight reduction—it is doubtful to turn on a 'thin quality' with nourishment." Moreover, while these "sirtfoods" are without a doubt substantial, large man-Roth says somebody would need to ensure they are additionally balancing their suppers with sound fats and proteins.

Concerning the structure of the eating routine, it may not be significant. However, Cording figures it could be an agreeable choice for individuals who are keen on a weight-reduction plan that has some structure and offers space for adaptability and customization. "I welcome that it's a 'diet of incorporation' versus one concentrated basically on limiting nourishments," she says. So, Cording concedes that the juice-substantial beginning piece of Phase One is a bit lower in calories than what she would regularly prescribe. Yet, the later stages, which incorporate an unhealthier objective and healthy nourishment, are, to some degree, increasingly economical.

Synopsis:

Nourishment is loaded with vitality, which permits you to do things like showering, practicing and relaxing.

It is an individual from the mustard or Brassicaceae, family, as is cabbage and Brussels grows. Potential advantages incorporate overseeing circulatory strain, boosting stomach related wellbeing, and ensuring against malignant growth and type 2 diabetes.

Advantages:

Devouring kale may help support stomach related wellbeing, among different benefits. Kale contains fiber, cancer prevention agents, calcium, nutrients C and K, iron, and a full scope of different supplements that can help forestall various medical issues.

Cancer prevention agents help the body expel undesirable poisons that outcome from diagnostic procedures and ecological weights. These poisons, known as free radicals, are unsteady particles. On the off chance that too many developers in the body, they can prompt cell harm. This may bring about medical issues, for example, irritation and ailments. Specialists accept that free radicals may assume a job in the advancement of the disease, for instance.

Diabetes:

The American Diabetes Association suggests devouring nourishments that are plentiful in nutrients, minerals, fiber, and cancer prevention agents. There is proof that a portion of these may offer security against diabetes.

Fiber: A recent report presumed that individuals who devour the most elevated measures of dietary fiber seem to have a lower danger of creating type 2 diabetes. Eating dietary fiber may likewise bring down blood glucose levels, the creators note.

Cell reinforcements: Authors of a 2012 article note that high glucose levels can trigger the generation of free radicals. They note that cancer prevention agents, for example, nutrient C and alpha-linolenic corrosive (ALA), can help lessen entanglements that may happen with diabetes. Both of these cancer prevention agents are available in kale.

Coronary illness:

Different supplements in kale may bolster heart wellbeing.

Potassium: The American Heart Association (AHA) prescribes expanding the admission of potassium while decreasing the utilization of included salt, or sodium. This, states the AHA, can diminish the danger of hypertension and cardiovascular sickness. A cup of cooked kale gives 3.6% of a grown-up's everyday requirements for potassium.

Fiber: Individuals who consumed more fiber were bound to have lower levels of total cholesterol and low-thickness lipoprotein (LDL) or "awful" cholesterol. Individuals need both dissolvable and insoluble fiber.

Kale and green vegetables that contain chlorophyll can help keep the body from engrossing heterocyclic amines. These synthetic compounds happen when individuals flame broil creature determined nourishments at a high temperature. Specialists have connected them with malignancy.

The human body cannot assimilate a lot of chlorophyll; however, chlorophyll ties to these cancer-causing agents and keeps the body from retaining them.

Cell reinforcements: Nutrient C, beta carotene, selenium, and different cell reinforcements in kale may help forestall disease. Studies have not discovered that enhancements have a similar impact. Yet, individuals who have a high admission of foods grown from the ground seem to have a lower danger of creating different tumors. This might be because of the cell reinforcements these nourishments contain.

Fiber: A high utilization of fiber may help decrease the danger of colorectal disease, as indicated by an investigation from 2015.

Bone wellbeing:

Calcium and phosphorus are pivotal for sound bone development. Some examination has recommended that a high admission of nutrient K may help decrease the danger of bone cracks. A cup of cooked kale gives just about multiple times a grown-up's daily requirement for nutrient K, around 18% of their calcium need, and about 7% of the day by day phosphorus necessity.

Absorption

Kale is high in fiber and water, the two of which help forestall obstruction and advance normality and a stable stomach related tract.

Skin and hair

Kale is a decent wellspring of beta-carotene, the carotenoid that the body changes over into nutrient an as it needs it. Beta-carotene and nutrient are essential for the development and support of all body tissues, including the skin and hair. The body utilizes nutrient C to fabricate and look after collagen, a protein that gives structure to skin, hair, and bones. Nutrient C is likewise present in kale. A cup of cooked kale offers at any rate 20% of an individual's day by day requirement for nutrient An and over 23% of the day by day necessity for nutrient C.

Eye wellbeing

Kale contains lutein and zeaxanthin, a cell reinforcement blend that may help decrease the danger of old enough related macular degeneration. Nutrient C, nutrient E, beta-carotene, and zinc additionally assume a job in eye wellbeing. These are available in kale.

Red Wine as Diet food

Research shows that resveratrol, a fixing found in grapes, berries and red wine can help transform fat into calorie-consuming 'dark-colored' fat. Simply drink capably! ... They found that in spite of a high-fat eating routine, the mice put on 40% less weight than creatures did not bolster the compound.

Wine darlings celebrate! Research has demonstrated that fixing in grapes, berries and red wine can transform abundance fat into calorie-consuming "dark colored" fat. The revelation proposes that diets containing the substance, resveratrol, may help battle weight. Researchers gave mice measures of resveratrol identical to people devouring 12 ounces of organic product every day. They found that in spite of a high-fat eating regimen, the mice put on 40% less weight than creatures did not bolster the compound.

Starting to eat better used to mean removing every "awful" nourishment and beverages to get in shape, and liquor was commonly the first to go. In addition to the fact that it adds additional calories, yet it likewise makes it simpler to store carbs as fat as opposed to consuming them off. Be that as it may, for some, an individual, adhering to an eating plan that restricts alcohol is not just unsavory and troublesome, yet additionally probably not going to be feasible for long haul objectives.

Chapter 5: Sirtfood Diet – Phase 1

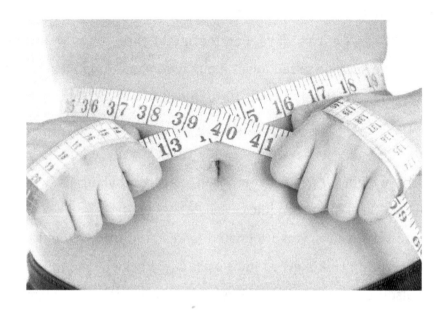

The plan asserts that eating particular foods can trigger your "lean receptor" pathway and possess you losing seven pounds in seven days. Foods such as ginseng, dark chocolate, and milk contain a natural compound called polyphenols which mimic the results of fasting and exercise. Strawberries, red onions, cinnamon, and garlic will also be powerful sirtfoods. These foods can activate the sirtuin pathway to help activate weight reduction. The science seems appealing, however, in reality, there is very little research to support these claims. Plus, the guaranteed speed of weight reduction from the very first week is quite quick and perhaps not in accord with the National Institute of Health safe fat loss recommendations of a couple of pounds each week.

This phase includes 2 phases:

Phase 1 lasts for two days. For the initial three days, you only drink three sirtfood green juices along with something meal full of sirtfoods for an overall total of 1000 calories.

Phase 2 is really a 14day maintenance program, though it is created to your shed weight steadily (perhaps not maintain your present weight). Daily is composed of three balanced sirtfood meals plus also one green juice.

After those 3 weeks, you are invited to keep on eating a diet full of sirtfoods and drink a green juice each day. Buckwheat and lovage may also be things that can be encouraged for use in your green juice. The diet urges that juices need to be prepared by a juicer, so perhaps not really a blender, so that it tastes better.

Now, you absolutely will need to plan and also have access to the ingredients that are recommended in order to correctly stick to this diet program. You can also have to put money into an adequate juicer, which can set you back no less than $100.

The seasonality of components makes it somewhat tough to have kale and tomatoes times of this season. Additionally, it is hard to follow if traveling at social events and feeding a family with young children.

Sirtfood Diet-Phase 1

The diet cuts numerous food collections and also it is limiting. Dairy foods that give a range of crucial nutritional elements including several that a lot of folk's lack, is not advocated in the strategy. What is more, the polyphenol-rich food Matcha frequently contains lead from the tea leaves that will be potentially dangerous for your health particularly when taken regularly. Additionally, it includes a robust and bitter flavor, as doe's 85% black chocolate which is also suggested.

What is your Sirtfood diet?

Creators of that sirtfood diet say that foods full of polyphenols (antioxidants) influence "lean" genes inside the human body which mimic fasting and exercise, jumpstart weight reduction, promote metabolism, boost mood, and enhance aging. Cases of polyphenol-rich foods that the sirtfood diet encourages you to eat comprise of green tea extract, black chocolate, green, red wine, as well as kale.

Sirtfood nutrition strategies

When you abide by the sirtfood daily diet, you are going to start out with Phase 1 – that lasts for two days. Throughout the first 3 days of this daily diet plan, you are to drink three sirtfood juices and also consume just one sirtfood-rich meal to get a regular total of 1000 calories.

Phase 2 lasts a fortnight and enables one to eat three balanced sirtfood-rich meals plus also one green juice each day. Once Phase 2 is finished, you are going to adhere to a more ordinary manner of eating – however, you are encouraged to include sirtuin-activating foods to routine meal plans. It is possible to re-enter Phase 1 and 2 any moment you will need to shed weight or excess fat.

Foods you may eat

You will probably wish to get a juicer before beginning the sirtfood diet. These foods and beverages are supported:

- Green juices (including Matcha green tea extract, lovage, and buckwheat)
- Green tea
- Coffee
- Cocoa powder
- Dark chocolate
- Beef
- Kale
- Onions
- Parsley
- Coffee
- Coconut oil
- Crimson chicory
- Noodle berry
- Berries
- Walnuts
- Eggs
- Bacon
- Turkey
- Seafood
- Whole grain pitas
- Cheese
- Hummus
- Buckwheat noodles
- Red wine

Avoid milk-based foods when on the sirtfood diet plan.

Does the diet work?

One reason you will probably lose some pounds in the event that you adhere to it is because the sirtfood diet works since you'll reduce calories (at least in Phase 1) to 1,000 to 1,500 calories every day, which can be an almost sure-fire method to lose weight. The main point is that you never need to eat sirtuin-activating foods to lose weight (simply lowering your current calories will have the desired effect), however, nearly all sirtfoods are healthier, seem to reduce disease risks, and also help with healthy weight control.

Phase 1:

This last for seven days plus, it is divided up. Throughout the first three days, you should consume three sirtfood green juices and also a routine meal which is full of sirtfoods – for an overall total of 1000 calories each day.

To start with, science fiction. Sirtuins -- by which sirt has its own name -- really are some set of silent information regulator (Sir) proteins which increase our metabolic rate, boost muscle efficacy, turn on fat burning procedures, reduce redness and repair damage. In conclusion, sirtuins allow us to become thinner and fitter (additionally, there are signs that they may possibly help combat acute diseases like Alzheimer's and diabetes.

Mild forms of stress – for example, exercise and calorie restriction – activate the system's production of sirtuins, however, it has been discovered that chemical substances called sirtuin activators, found naturally in vegetables and fruit, may perform exactly the very same task. Food items – sirtfoods, since they will have been consumed by dietary plan producers – are notably saturated in those sirtuin activators and thus, the theory goes, even should you eat a diet chiefly made up of these food items, and you'll reduce weight and enhance your wellbeing.

To test this thought, Goggins and Matten established the sirt diet, the seven-day eating program that caused all of the fuss. It is simple enough: throughout the first 3 days, daily caloric consumption is limited by 1000 and is made up of three orange juices, and a sirtfood-rich beverage. On four to seven, calories are raised to 1,500 and are made up of two juices along with two meals. After that all-out very first week, your recommendation would be to eat a balanced diet full of sirtfoods, combined side an increase of green juices. On the surface of it, that sounds bad: most fasting diet plans allow greater calories. However, can it be?

I did not really feel hard done whatsoever," states Rannoch Donald, a trainer that tried this diet program. "The juice is vital: it's like rocket fuel. After the first week, then following the diet has been plain sailing, after three weeks that I became 5kg lighter. But crucially, I felt that the best that I have in a few years. I lost body fat, so I had been sleeping, I would no stomach difficulties, I had been feeling caked... I had been training and teaching half of a dozen classes weekly with fantastic healing, even by the very grueling Brazilian jiujitsu session."

To examine the dietary plan on a broader scale. We had been performing a moderate quantity of exercise; none increased it plus some began doing. And the consequences in only a single week considering the calorie limitation were astonishing: that the evaluation subjects lost on average 3kg of fat however placed on approximately 0.8kilogram of muscle. With a normal diet which cut off calories at precisely the exact same amount in each week, you would be expecting to eliminate a max of 1kg.

How do I prepare for your initial phase of this daily diet?

It is the clear question: should sirtuins are therefore game-changing, why are not pharmaceutical and nutritional supplement organizations attempting to distill them in pill form? Short answer: since the mechanics whereby they operate are still not fully known, meaning supplements will not necessarily function if absorbed from your system as the organic forms.

In supplement form, it is poorly consumed by the entire human anatomy, however, in its own normal food matrix of red wine, its bioavailability (just how much your human body is able to utilize) is six-fold greater. We believe it's much better to eat up a vast selection of these nutritional elements from the kind of pure whole foods, where they revolve together with the countless of additional natural bioactive plant compounds that act responsibly to enhance our wellness." Other words, instead of simply popping a pill.

Fast and mad?

Obviously, this really is the component of this sirt diet that is critiqued. Most importantly out of this simple fact, at least at the beginning phases, the master plan is targeted on calorie restriction also that, in accordance with previous adventure, weight loss over 1kg per week is either poor or unsustainable. This is really a legal concern: in many calorie restriction food diets, premature weight reduction has a tendency to stem in calorie depletion and paid off water-bloating, and as recent research about contestants at television's the biggest loser shows – only rationing yourself each single day can slow your metabolic rate to some near-permanent crawl, and in addition to messing with the levels of "hunger hormone" ghrelin, which makes you eternally famished.

However, this is simply not exactly what sirt does. Yes, even this diet mimics some facets of fasting, also in the very initial seven days of the complete diet sirtfoods may actually turbocharge the effects of calorie restriction. However, it is a little more complex compared to simply starving for short-term alterations. Just how can this work? Well, firstly, it is crucial to know the "stress" part of this equation. Everybody needs a certain quantity of stress in their own lives. Every single time we train we produce pressure in your human anatomy, which is a fantastic thing or something. There is a temptation to always train tougher, to strive harder, however that conveys a probability to build up chronic stress, which includes the chance of overtraining along with a diminished immune system."

The flip side: by exposing your own body to low-grade sources of stress, you are going to raise the ability to deal with it. Plant pressure reactions are now more complicated compared to our own. Think of it: if we are thirsty and hungry, we could proceed in hunt of food and beverage; overly hot – we find shade; under attack – we are able to flee. In comparison, plants have been stationary and have to survive every one of the extremes of the physiological pressures and dangers. As a result, in the last billion decades, they've developed an extremely sophisticated stress-response system which lowers stress by creating a vast selection of organic plant compounds -- known as polyphenols -- which let them successfully adjust to their own environment and survive. When we eat these crops, we also eat this polyphenol nourishment that triggers our own inborn stress-response pathways. We are talking here in the exact very same pathways of fasting and physical exercise and both switch on the sirtuins.

Chapter 6: Sirtfood Diet – Phase 2

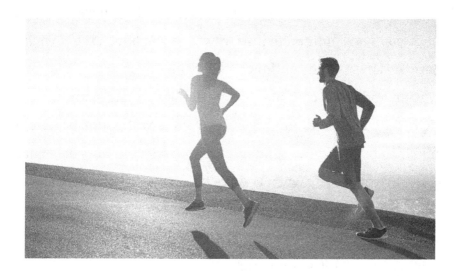

Once you have made it to the second phase you no longer have to count calories. Your reset week is over and now you simply have to maintain you are new, more healthful habits. From this point forward, your meals should be celebrations of the food you are consuming.

The goal of the Sirtfood Diet is to set you up for lifelong success incorporating these nutrient-dense sirtfoods into your daily life. The maintenance phase is a 2-week period to help you transition from your previous diet, beyond the dietary reset and into an eating routine that is founded on health.

During Phase 2, your commitment is going to be dedicated to finding a routine that fits nicely into your unique lifestyle. You want to create habits of health so that your daily food decisions become easier and more automatic over time, with sirtfoods being the natural solution to your hunger.

Even though you are no longer counting calories, there is a good chance you will continue to lose weight, if you have excess weight to lose. As long as you continue to enjoy plenty of sirtfoods in your life, your body will continue to find its health and natural, ideal weight. As your health improves, your body will better be able to communicate with you, sending you more stable hunger signals and telling you clearly when you are full.

During the next 2 weeks, you are encouraged to start your day refreshed with a green juice and then balance your metabolism smoothly with 3 full, sirtfood rich meals.

Nutrient Density

As you start to return, you're eating habits back to a more consistent 3 meals per day, your primary focus should be on making sure that the majority of foods that make it to your plate are chosen for their nutritional content. Most important, their polyphenol content.

Phase 2 is not about counting calories, but you should still be aware of how much you are feeding your body. Portion sizes have become drastically disproportionate to our health needs in recent years, so it may take a bit of experimentation to find your own, personal healthy balance.

A really key component of healthy eating is setting time aside during your day to focus, specifically on eating. Pay attention to your food instead of rushing to eat as quickly as possible before running out the door or eating mindlessly as you watch television. In both circumstances, you are not allowing your body to decide how much food it needs, which more often than not leads to overeating. If instead, you sit down with friends or family, or even quietly by yourself, and pay attention to the process of eating, your body will give you cues when it is starting to fill up.

The Japanese have a mantra that they repeat before each meal: hara hachi bu. It is an ancient Confucian saying that reminds you to eat only until you are 80% full. This is very wise because it can take some time for your brain to realize your stomach is full. By the time you think you are full, you are probably already past this point.

As you learn how to listen to your biological hunger cues again, your taste buds will also be going through a natural adjustment period. They will need to re-learn what real, healthy food should taste like. You will be surprised at how quickly your tastes will change, but as a general rule, you need to introduce a new few approximately 7 times before you will really learn to enjoy it. These next 2 weeks are designed to prove to you that, when you put your mind to it, you can learn to love healthy foods that are going to love your body in return.

Getting comfortable in your kitchen, if you are not already, is going to make a big difference in your life. It is a good idea to get familiar with some of the ingredients that are going to become staples in your home from now on.

Two more ingredients that should be fairly easy to incorporate into a wide variety of meals, and easily find at almost any grocery store, are arugula, also known as rocket, and kale. For many years, spinach has been the leafy green to swap into your meals, but it is time to mix it up. Spinach is packed with nutrition and even polyphenols, but arugula and kale provide new flavors and textures for you to try, and also more variety in types of polyphenols. Just like you need a wide variety of vitamins, from A to K, so too will you be at your healthiest with a variety of polyphenols. So, mix up your leafy greens, but always try to reach for the richest, darkest shades of green.

You can use greens in many different ways, so they are a highly versatile vegetable to always have in good supply in your fridge. You can, of course, add greens to your juice in the morning, and use them for the obvious salads and sandwich fillers. But great leafy vegetables are also delicious sautéed with a bit of olive oil and garlic or added to your buckwheat pasta dishes. Arugula has a spicy flavor and delicate leaves, whereas kale is woodier and brings a lot of texture to your dish, a good reminder to put your saliva to work as you chew your food well before swallowing. You can even sirtify your snack time; kale chips are a surprisingly simple treat to toast up in just a few minutes.

Focusing on adding more variety of leafy greens to your meals is a simple solution to increase the nutrient density of your food but getting familiar with herbs and spices can bring even more variety to your meals.

Hot chili peppers, garlic, and parsley are probably all relatively familiar to you, but turmeric might not be as frequently used in your kitchen, though hopefully, it will be in your future.

If you have ever enjoyed Indian food, you have most likely had turmeric. This spice is one of the well-researched foods on earth, and it has been used in traditional medicines for thousands of years. Thanks to a phytochemical called curcumin, it is a natural anti-inflammatory agent that is very well known for its antioxidant capacity. It also happens to be very good at activating sirtuins.

Turmeric is widely used in Indian cuisine; responsible for the bright yellow hue of many curries, but it has a surprisingly mild flavor, making it suitable to add to a wide variety of dishes. Add a pop of color to your juices or smoothies, soups, stews, grain, or pasta dishes, and it even makes a relaxing and delicious tea.

When you are planning your meals, it is important that you think beyond the focal ingredients and look for ways to add more sirtfoods, either as filler ingredients or even spices. Any extra sirtfood will increase the nutrient-density of your meals.

Digesting Sirtfoods

The more we learn about the health of our microbiome, or gut, the more obvious it is that it is a keystone to our overall health and enjoyment of life.

Many people are forced to plan their daily activities around the availability and accessibility of a toilet. This is not a happy or comfortable situation to be in but having a healthy digestive system can impact more than just your daily bowel movements, however distressing they may be.

There is more and more evidence flooding the medical scene that shows how closely related our gut is to both our immune system and our brain health. Autoimmune disorders are on the rise, affecting millions of people in the USA alone. Bacterial infections that begin in your microbiome can directly affect learning and memory, and long-term intestinal damage can significantly increase your risk of cognitive decline.

When researchers looked very closely at the communication patterns between the gut and the brain, it turns out that only 10% of the messages start in the brain, usually during a stress response when the brain suggests the gut stops working temporarily so that energy can be put to better use elsewhere. In fact, if this happens and there is a lot of undigested food in waiting, your body may try to get rid of it quickly to save resources, and you could find yourself experiencing nervous vomiting or diarrhea in very stressful situations.

The other 90% of the communication, however, is traveling from our gut to our brain. This is logical, though it sometimes comes as a surprise to people. Your gut has more square footage that your entire skin does, so it is responsible for the intake of a lot of information about our nutritional status. It knows everything about what we are, or are not, feeding it in terms of nutrition. It is also responsible for training our entire immune system. If our brain needs information about our health, the first place it asks is our gut.

It makes sense then that people who suffer from chronic digestive distress are going to be more at risk for diseases of the brain and mental health disorders.

The health of your gut depends on keeping a thriving community of healthy bacteria.

When you eat food, it gets digested in many phases, starting with your saliva, and ending up in a mixture of highly acidic stomach juices. If this digestive process does not successfully break all the food particles down into their simplest components, you will start to have trouble with the absorption of the nutrients from the food. Sometimes, food particles that are only partially broken down will find their way into our bloodstream, where they can do damage and lead to an overactive autoimmune system. This is often called "leaky gut syndrome." Other times, we simply will not absorb the nutrition and we will miss out on the value of the food we are eating.

To help make sure our food is properly digested, massive colonies of healthy bacteria line our entire digestive tract but primarily live in our intestines and colon. They feed on components of our food that we cannot break down effectively, particularly fiber, which creates a symbiotic relationship between the bacteria and our gut.

Foods that feed these helpful bacteria are called prebiotics and primarily consist of specific kinds of fiber. Some common examples are garlic, onions and legumes or beans. Your body does not digest the fiber in these foods very well, but they are enjoyed as the favorite nutrition source for the bacteria instead.

Certain types of food can also hurt and even kill the good bacteria in your microbiome. Flooding your gut with too much sugar and unhealthy fats will encourage the growth of harmful bacteria that, in time, can outnumber your good bacteria. Studies also show that some of the poisons that are used in conventional farming practices will not just kill the bugs that eat fresh produce, but it will also kill the bacteria in your gut.

Finally, antibiotics, though incredibly useful in killing harmful and potentially deadly bacterial infections, do not discriminate and will also kill healthy bacteria. If you ever need a course of antibiotics, one of the best things you can do for your long-term health is to follow this treatment with plenty of probiotic foods and possibly even supplements, to help repopulate your gut with good bacteria.

You may be wondering where these healthy bacteria come from in the first place though. They are introduced through specific foods as well: probiotics.

Chapter 7: Sirtfood For Life - Sustainability and Benefits

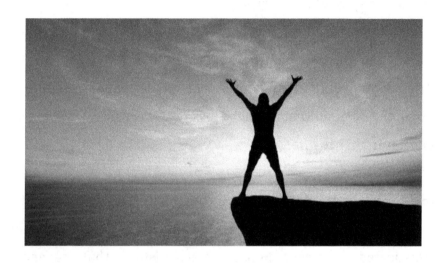

You have entered the hyper-success process, achieving weight loss in the area of 7 pounds, which probably includes an attractive increase in muscle. You also maintained your weight loss throughout the fourteen-day maintenance phase and further strengthened the body composition. Perhaps notably, you have marked the beginning of your transformation of wellness. You took a stand against the tide of ill health, which strikes as often as we get older. The life you have decided for yourself is enhanced strength, productivity, and health.

By now, you will be familiar with the top twenty Sirtfoods, and you have gained a sense of how powerful they are. Not only that, you will probably have become quite good at including them in your diet and loving them. For the sustained weight loss and health, they offer, these items must stay a prominent feature in your everyday eating regimen. But still, they are just twenty foods, and after all, the spice of life is variety.

It is about getting your body in perfect balance with a diet that is suitable and sustainable for everyone and providing all the nutrients we need that enhance our health. It is about keeping on reaping the Sirtfood Diet's weight-loss rewards using the very best foods nature has to offer.

Some other Sirtfoods

We have seen why Sirtfoods are so beneficial: certain plants have sophisticated stress-response mechanisms that generate compounds that trigger sirtuins— the same fasting and exercise-activated fat-burning and durability mechanism in the body. The greater the quantity of these compounds generated by plants in response to stress, the greater the value we derive from their feeding. Our list of the top twenty Sirtfoods is made up of the foods that stand out because they are particularly packed full of these compounds, and hence the foods that have the most exceptional ability to impact body composition and wellbeing. But foods ' sirtuin-activating results aren't a concept of all or nothing. There are many other plants out there that produce moderate levels of sirtuin-activating nutrients, and by eating these liberally, we encourage you to expand the variety and diversity of your diet. The Sirtfood Diet is all about inclusion and the greater the range of sirtuin-activating items that can be integrated into the diet. Especially if that means you will obtain from your meals even more of your favorite foods to increase pleasure and enjoyment.

Let us use the workout comparison. The top twenty Sirtfoods are the (much more pleasurable) equivalent of sweating it out at the gym, with Phase 1 being the "boot camp." By contrast, eating those other foods with more moderate levels of sirtuin-activating nutrients is like reaping the rewards of going out for a good walk. Contrast that to the typical diet that has a nutritional value equal to sitting all day on the couch watching Television. Yeah, sweating it out in the gym is fine, but if that is all you do, you will quickly get fed up with it. The walk should also be welcomed, especially if it means that you do not just choose to sit on the sofa.

For e.g., in our top twenty Sirtfoods, we have included strawberries because they are the most prominent source of the sirtuin activator fisetin. Yet if we look more broadly at berries as a food group, we find that they have metabolic health benefits as well as healthy ageing. Reviewing their nutritional content, we note that other berries such as blackberries, black currants, blueberries, and raspberries also have significant amounts of nutrients that cause sirtuins.

The same holds with nuts. Notwithstanding their calorific material, nuts are so effective that they promote weight loss and help shift inches from the waist. This is in addition to cutting chronic disease risk. Though walnuts are our champion nut, nutrients that trigger sirtuin can also be found in chestnuts, pecans, pistachios, and even peanuts.

Instead, we turn our attention to food. Throughout recent years there has been in several areas an increasing aversion to grains. Studies, however, link whole grain consumption with decreased inflammation, diabetes, heart disease, and cancer. Although they do not equal the pseudo-grain buckwheat Sirtfood qualifications, we do see the existence of substantial sirtuin-activating nutrients in other whole grains. And needless to say, their sirtuin-activating nutrient quality is decimated when whole grains are converted into refined "clean" forms. Such modified models are quite dangerous groups and are interested in a number of state-of-the-art health problems. We are not saying you can never eat them, but instead, you are going to be much better off sticking to the whole-grain version whenever possible.

With the likes of goji berries and chia seeds possessing Sirtfood powers, also notorious "superfoods" get on the bandwagon. That is most likely the unwitting reason for the health benefits they have observed. While it does imply that they are healthy for us to consume, we do know that there are easier, more available, and better options out there, so do not feel compelled to get on that specific bandwagon! We see the same trend across a lot of food categories. Unsurprisingly, the foods that research has developed are usually good for us, and we should be consuming more of them.

Power of Protein

A high protein diet is one of the most popular diets of the last few years. Higher protein intake while dieting has been shown to encourage satiety, sustain metabolism, and reduce muscle mass loss. But it is when they pair Sirtfoods with protein that things get brought to a whole new level. Protein is, as you may remember, a necessary addition in a diet based on Sirtfood to gain maximum benefits. Protein consists of amino acids, and it is a particular amino acid, leucine, which effectively complements Sirtfoods ' behavior, strengthening their effects. This is done primarily by changing our cellular environment so that our diet's sirtuin-activating nutrients work much more effectively. It ensures we get the best result from a Sirtfood-rich meal, which is paired with protein-based in leucine. Leucine's main dietary sources contain red meat, pork, fruit, vegetables, milk, and dairy products.

Animal Based-Protein

Animal products have been implicated in recent years as a contributing cause of many Western diseases, especially cancer. If that is the case, eating them with Sirtfoods may not sound like such a bright idea. Here is our lowdown to lay that to rest.

One of the significant concerns regarding milk is that it is not just a simple food but a highly sophisticated signaling mechanism to cause rapid offspring body production. Although this has a cherished meaning in early life, it may not be so common in adult life. Persistent and hyper activating the primary growth signal now correlated with ageing and the progression of age-related disorders such as obesity, type 2 diabetes, cancer, and neurodegenerative diseases. Notwithstanding the intricacies of this signaling system being a relatively new area of research and thus still very much an uncertain and theoretical possibility, this does explain why people might shy away from dairy products. However, the study points to one thing: if we add Sirtfoods to a dairy-containing diet, they inhibit mTOR's inappropriate effects on our cells, rescind this risk, making Sirtfoods a must-include with a dairy-based diet.

Generally, there are mixed reviews of the association between dairy and cancer. If we stack up all the study, mild dairy consumption is perfectly fine in the sense of a Sirtfood-rich diet and can deliver several useful nutrients to supplement Sirtfoods.

Poultry is ok when it comes to meat and cancer risk, but red and fried meats are much more suspect. Although data concerning them in breast and prostate cancer on the field is pretty thin, there is a legitimate concern that red and processed meat eating plays a role in intestinal cancer. Processed meat, such as sausages tends to be the worst perpetrator. Although there is no need to take it off the table, it should be included in just small amounts, rather than being a constant.

The good news for red meat is that research shows that cooking it with Sirtfoods rescues the risk of cancer, whether it's making a marinade with herbs, seasoning, and extra virgin olive oil; frying the beef with onions, or simply adding a nice cup of green tea to the meal or indulging in dark chocolate after dinner.

These all pack a punch from Sirtfood, which helps to neutralize the harmful effects of red meat. While we are all out to have the steak and consume it, do not go crazy. Red meat consumption is best kept at around 1 pound (500 g) per week (cooked weight), roughly equivalent to 1.5 pounds (700 to 750 g) fresh.

The link between egg consumption and cancer risk has not been investigated as extensively as meat and dairy products have, but there seems little cause for concern in this regard. Which eggs have been active in inducing is heart disease, instead? This is because they constitute a significant dietary cholesterol source. Thus, we are advised to restrict the use of eggs. Further countries, including Nepal, benefit interestingly. Who is right, then? The reason for siding with the latter is compelling. There is no linked routine egg intake with any increased risk of coronary heart disease or stroke. Although specific genetic disorders that involve a decreased consumption of dietary cholesterol, this limitation is not appropriate for the general population.

The Power of Three

The omega-3 long-chain fatty acids EPA and DHA are the second major category of nutrients that effectively complement Sirtfoods. Omega-3s have been the coveted natural wellbeing global favorite for years. What we did not know before, which we are doing now, is that they also improve the activation of a group of sirtuin genes in the body that is directly linked to longevity. It makes them the perfect match for Sirtfoods.

Omega-3s have potent effects in decreasing inflammation and lowering fat blood levels. To that, we can add additional heart-healthy effects: rendering the blood less likely to pool, stabilizing the heart's electrical activity, and lowering blood pressure. Even the pharmaceutical industry now looks to them as an aid in the war against cardiac disease. And that is not where the litany of benefits ends. Omega-3s also have an effect on the way we perceive, having been shown to boost the outlook and help stave off dementia.

When we speak about omega-3s, we are thinking primarily about eating fish, particularly oily types, because no other dietary source comes close to supplying the significant levels of EPA and DHA that we need. And to see the benefits, all we need is two servings of fish a week, with an emphasis on oily fish. Sadly, the United States is not a country of big fish eaters, and that is accomplished by less than one in five Americans. As a result, our intake of the precious EPA and DHA is appallingly short.

Plant foods, including almonds, beans, and green leafy vegetables, often produce omega-3 but in a form called alpha-linolenic acid, which must be processed into EPA or DHA in the body. This conversion process is poor, meaning that alpha-linolenic acid delivers a negligible amount of our needs for omega-3. Even with the wonderful advantages of Sirtfoods, we should not forget the added value that drinking adequate omega-3 fats provide. In that order, the best sources of omega-3 fish are herring, sardines, salmon, trout, and mackerel. While fresh tuna is naturally high, too, the tinned version loses the majority of the omega 3. And a replacement of DHA-enriched microalgae (up to 300 milligrams a day) is also recommended for vegetarians and vegans, though food foods should still be integrated into the diet.

Chapter 8: Questions and Answers

Amanda is a Healthy Food Guide's nourishment manager with a degree in sustenance and a post-graduate recognition in dietetics. She is an individual from the British Dietetic Association, The Nutrition Society and The Guild of Food...

Eat chocolate, drink red wine, and get thinner? Amanda Upsell investigates the current year's most overwhelming eating regimen plan

The Sirtfood Diet by Aidan Goggin's and Glen Matten (both of whom have a boss's degree in wholesome drug) guarantees you will lose 7lb in seven days. Numerous VIPs are, obviously, lapping it up. Would it be advisable for us to do likewise?

What is the reason?

It depends on eating a gathering of nourishments that contain something the creators portray as 'sirtuin activators'. Sirtuins are a class of protein, seven of which (SIRT1 to SIRT7) have been recognized in people. They seem to have a wide scope of jobs in our body, including potential enemies of maturing and metabolic impacts.

As researchers see increasingly about sirtuins, they are getting keen on the job they may play in assisting with turning on those weight reduction pathways that are normally activated by an absence of nourishment and by taking activity. The hypothesis goes that in the event that you can actuate a portion of the seven sirtuins, you could assist with consuming fat and treat weight with less exertion than it takes to follow some different eating regimens or go through hours on the treadmill.

What does it include?

The Sirtfood Diet has two phases. On every one of the initial three days, you drink three 'sirt juices' and have one supper (aggregate of 1,000 calories per day). On the accompanying four days, you are permitted two sirt juices and two dinners day by day (aggregate of 1,500 calories day by day). You at that point progress to the simpler stage two, with one juice and three 'adjusted' dinners, in reasonable bit measures, a day.

What would you be able to eat on the eating regimen?

There is a rundown of nourishments containing synthetic intensifies that the creators' state switches on sirtuin and wrench up fat consumption while at the same time bringing down hunger (the last most likely through assisting with accomplishing better glucose control).

Is it compelling for weight reduction?

You ought to get in shape essentially on the grounds that you are eating fewer calories, particularly in stage one. Without a doubt, you may consume fat quicker with this eating routine than with 'any old calorie-confined' plan and you may feel fuller. With respect to the creators' case, this eating regimen is 'clinically demonstrated to lose 7lb in seven days'...

Indeed, it is important that so far, the eating regimen has just been tried on 40 sound, exceptionally energetic human guinea pigs in an upmarket rec center in London's Knightsbridge. The analyzers lost a normal of 7lb in seven days while demonstrating increments in bulk and vitality. In any case, at that point given the calorie limitations of that first week, weight reduction may essentially be because of the extraordinary decrease in calories.

The decision

Further examinations are expected to distinguish the long-haul sway on waistlines – and general wellbeing – and to see whether sirt calorie counters keep the pounds off any more adequately than they would on different eating regimens. We do not yet have the foggiest idea what, assuming any, sway the expansion of Sirt foods to our eating regimen really has on our weight.

What is more, will anybody have the option to stay with the repetitiveness of juices and limit themselves to nourishments on the rundown (and be glad to dump their typical cuppa for green tea) for all time? With respect to the features that recommend you can appreciate dull chocolate and red wine on this eating regimen – well, truly, it is anything but a green light to expend piles of either!

Cutting calories will consistently give you results

In the event that you have the funds, the tendency, and the stomach for it, I am very certain it will 'attempt' somewhat for the time being, if simply because it is a successful method to confine calories. Furthermore, wine and chocolate aside, the rundown, for the most part, comprises of the very nourishments dietitians and nutritionists suggest for good wellbeing (think products of the soil!).

Regardless of whether it functions admirably enough to make it stand separated from a huge number of weight reduction designs that have trodden this tired way before likewise is not yet clear.

Chapter 9: Sirtfood Recipes

No Added Sugar Granola

Preparation Time: 30 minutes

Cooking Time: 30 minutes

Servings: 6

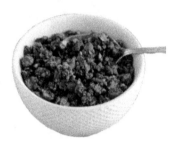

INGREDIENTS
- 1 ½ cups rolled oats
- 1 ½ cups buckwheat groats, r:
- ½ cup walnuts, chopped
- ½ cup slivered almonds
- ½ cup sunflower seeds
- 2 cups shredded coconut
- 1 cup Medjool dates, chopped
- 1 cup raisins
- ¼ cup dark chocolate chips or chunks (at least 85%)
- 1/4 cup extra virgin olive oil
- 1 cup water

For serving (optional):
- 1 cup milk or yogurt

DIRECTIONS

1. This recipe has sugar in it, which is important to note for anyone following a sugar-free diet, but it is all natural and in stark contrast to the store-bought granola that is heavily laden with high-fructose corn syrup and other added

sugars. This granola is even more flavorful and delicious, and completely devoid of added sugar.
2. Preheat the oven to 350 degrees F.
3. In a small pot over medium heat, combine the dates and water. Cook until the mixture forms a thick paste, stirring occasionally. Remove from heat and set aside.
4. In a large bowl, mix together the oats, buckwheat groats, walnuts, almonds, sunflower seeds, coconut, raisins, and chocolate.
5. Spread out in a thin layer onto a large baking sheet or multiple baking sheets, as required.
6. Bake for 8 - 10 minutes, or until lightly toasted
7. Transfer the mixture back into the bowl, and add the date paste and oil, mixing well to coat thoroughly.
8. Return to the baking sheet and bake for an additional 8 to 10 minutes, stirring occasionally.
9. Granola crisps further as it cools, so allow standing for at least 30 minutes before eating.
10. Store extra granola in an airtight container

NUTRITION: Calories: 202 kcal Total Fat: 8.1 g Saturated Fat: 0.9 g Cholesterol: 0 mg Sodium: 36 mg Total Carbs: 27 g Fiber: 3.8 g Sugar: 5.4 g Protein: 3.8 g

Fruit 'N' Nut Granola

Preparation Time: 10 minutes

Cooking Time: 1 hour and 30 minutes

Servings: 5

INGREDIENTS

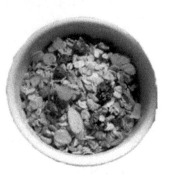

- 4 cups old-fashioned oats
- 1 cup buckwheat groats, raw
- 1 cup dry milk powder
- ½ cup Medjool dates, chopped
- 1 cup dried mixed fruit, chopped
- ½ cup walnuts, chopped
- ½ cup raw mixed nuts, chopped
- 1 tablespoon ground cinnamon
- ¾ cups packed brown sugar
- ¼ cup water
- ½ cup coconut oil, melted
- 1 teaspoon vanilla extract

DIRECTIONS

1. While very similar to the last recipe, this granola mix gives you more individual providence to select the dried fruits and nuts of your choice. While strawberries and walnuts are on the Top 20 Sirtfood list, other berries, fruits, and nuts have valuable nutrition as well, and variety keeps your breakfast more interesting.

2. Preheat oven to 275 degrees F.
3. In a large bowl, combine oats, buckwheat groats, milk powder, dried fruit, and dates, chopped nuts, and cinnamon.
4. In a saucepan over medium heat, bring brown sugar and water to a boil. Remove from the heat; stir in oil and vanilla until mixed.
5. Pour over oat mixture and mix well to coat. Pour into a large baking pan.
6. Bake for 1 hour and 30 minutes, stirring occasionally
7. Granola crisps further as it cools, so allow standing for at least 30 minutes before eating.
8. Store extra granola in an airtight container

NUTRITION: Calories: 224 kcal Total Fat: 8.2 g Saturated Fat: 3.5 g Cholesterol: 0 mg Sodium: 0 mg Total Carbs: 31.4 g Fiber: 4.1 g Sugar: 0 g Protein: 4.2 g

Buckwheat Muesli

Preparation Time: 5 minutes

Cooking Time: 0 minute

Servings: 2

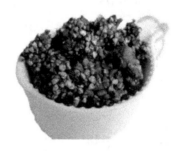

INGREDIENTS
- ¼ cup buckwheat flakes
- ¼ cup buckwheat puffs
- 1 tablespoon unsweetened desiccated coconut
- ¼ cup Medjool dates, chopped
- 1 tablespoon walnuts, chopped
- 1 teaspoon dark chocolate chips (at least 85%)

For Serving:
- ½ cup strawberries, chopped
- 1 cup milk or yogurt, as preferred

DIRECTIONS
1. The recipe can be doubled, or even quadrupled in order to store for future use. It is a simple combination that can be whipped up in a few minutes on your day off and used to fuel each morning of your week to come.
2. Mix all of the dry ingredients together.
3. Top with strawberries and serve with milk or yogurt.

NUTRITION: Calories: 218 kcal Total Fat: 10 g Saturated Fat: 2.7 g Cholesterol: 0 mg Sodium: 8 mg Total Carbs: 28 g Fiber: 3.1 g Sugar: 12 g Protein: 5.3 g

Strawberry Green Tea Oatmeal

Preparation Time: 10 minutes

Cooking Time: 0 minute

Servings: 4

INGREDIENTS
- 1 cup of strawberries, chopped
- 1 cup of oats
- ½ cup of milk
- ½ cup of green tea
- ¼ cup walnuts, crushed (optional)

DIRECTIONS
1. Cooking with green tea is a great way to add the health benefits of this incredible beverage to meals without any added effort. A green tea oatmeal will have slightly more depth to the flavor, but little other noticeable characteristics, beyond the benefits to your health.
2. Add green tea, oats, walnuts, and milk to a pot.
3. Stir over low heat until the oatmeal becomes thick (according to your package) and then remove the saucepan from heat.
4. Divide the oatmeal between 4 bowls and top with strawberries.

NUTRITION: Calories: 137 kcal Total Fat: 1 g Saturated Fat: 0 g Cholesterol: 0 mg Sodium: 0 mg Total Carbs: 29 g Fiber: 0 g Sugar: 0 g Protein: 2 g

Fluffy Vegan Pancakes

Preparation Time: 10 minutes

Cooking Time: 15 minutes

Servings: 8

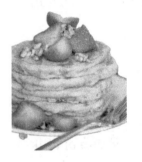

INGREDIENTS

- 1 very ripe banana, mashed
- ¾ cup soymilk
- 1 teaspoon extra virgin olive oil
- 1 teaspoon maple syrup (optional)
- 1 cup All-Purpose flour
- 1 ½ tablespoon baking powder

For serving (optional):

- 1 cup strawberries, quartered

DIRECTIONS

1. Pancakes are so simple to create and incredibly comforting to eat, the entire process should be cathartic. This vegan-friendly pancake batter will have built-in banana flavor, which is perfectly enhanced by a strawberry fruit topping.
2. Mash the banana well and add the milk, olive oil and maple syrup.
3. In a separate bowl, whisk together the flour, baking powder.

4. Add dry ingredients to wet ingredients and mix until well blended, but do not over mix.
5. Heat a lightly oiled griddle over medium-high heat. Drop batter onto the griddle in large spoonful's and cooks until lightly browned on the bottom. Watch for air bubbles. You will know it is time to flip your pancake when the air bubbles pop.
6. Flip your pancakes and cook until lightly browned on the other side. Repeat with remaining batter.
7. Serve topped with strawberries.

NUTRITION: Calories: 73.9 kcal Total Fat: 0.3 g Saturated Fat: 0.1 g Cholesterol: 0 mg Sodium: 383.2 mg Total Carbs: 15.8 g Fiber: 2.7 g Sugar: 1.8 g Protein: 3 g

Lentil, Kale, And Red Onion Pasta

Preparation Time: 10 minutes

Cooking Time: 35 minutes

Servings: 2

INGREDIENTS
- 2 ½ cups vegetable broth
- ¾ cup dry lentils
- 1 bay leaf
- ¼ cup olive oil
- 1 large red onion, chopped
- 1 teaspoon fresh thyme, chopped
- ½ teaspoon fresh oregano, chopped
- 8 ounces ground turkey, cut into ¼" slices (optional)
- 1 bunch kale, stems removed and leaves coarsely chopped
- 1 (12 ounce) package buckwheat pasta
- 2 tablespoons nutritional yeast
- Salt and pepper to taste

DIRECTIONS
1. If you cannot live without animal-based protein in your main dish, you can add some ground turkey or chicken, though be aware the lentils and pasta make this a hearty, protein packed dish without the need for meat.
2. Rinse the lentils in a fine mesh sieve under cold water until the water runs clear - this will prevent your lentils from getting gummy.

3. Bring the vegetable broth, lentils, ½ teaspoon of salt, and bay leaf to a boil in a saucepan over high heat. Reduce heat to medium-low, cover, and cook until the lentils are tender, about 20 minutes. Add additional broth if needed to keep the lentils moist. Discard the bay leaf once done.
4. As the lentils simmer, heat the olive oil in a skillet over medium-high heat. Stir in the onion, thyme, oregano, and season with salt and pepper to taste.
5. Cook for 1 minute, stirring often, then add the ground turkey, if using. Reduce the heat to medium-low, and cook until the onion has softened, about 10 minutes.
6. Meanwhile, bring a large pot of lightly salted water to a boil over high heat. Add the kale and pasta. Cook until the pasta is al dente, about 8 minutes.
7. Remove some of the cooking water and set aside. Drain the pasta, and then return to the pot.
8. Stir in the lentils, and onion mixture.
9. Use the reserved cooking liquid to adjust the sauciness of the dish to your liking. Sprinkle with nutritional yeast to serve

NUTRITION: Calories: 732 kcal Total Fat: 16.5 g Saturated Fat: 2 g Cholesterol: 0 mg Sodium: 1219 mg Total Carbs: 111.8 g Fiber: 19.3 g Sugar: 7 g Protein: 36.1 g

Arugula Linguine

Preparation Time: 10 minutes

Cooking Time: 25 minutes

Servings: 2

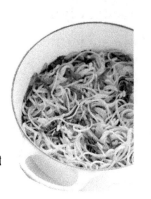

INGREDIENTS

- 12 ounces linguine or other dried past
- 3 tablespoons extra virgin olive oil
- 3 - 4 cloves garlic, sliced thinly
- 2 large handfuls baby arugula
- 2 tablespoons capers, drained
- ½ cup Parmesan, shredded or shaved
- 1/3 cup pine nuts, toasted

DIRECTIONS

1. Linguine is a light and fresh dish, perfect for a warm summer afternoon or evening, but the pasta also makes it appropriate for cooler times of year as well. The combination of capers, Parmesan and pine nuts is nothing short of magical.
2. Cook the pasta in a large pot of boiling salted water until al dente, about 8 minutes.
3. While pasta is cooking, heat oil in a large pan and sauté the garlic over medium heat for 2 – 3 minutes until just turning golden.

4. When your pasta is ready, drain and immediately add the remaining ingredients, including the garlic and toss to combine well.

NUTRITION: Calories: 188 kcal Total Fat: 8.2 g Saturated Fat: 1.1 g Cholesterol: 18.8 mg Sodium: 39.1 mg Total Carbs: 26.3 g Fiber: 3.2 g Sugar: 0.3 g Protein: 4.8 g

Potato Casserole

Preparation Time: 40 minutes

Cooking Time: 1 hour

Servings: 6 to 8

INGREDIENTS
For the Potato Crust:
- 5 russet potatoes, peeled
- 1 clove garlic, crushed
- 1 stalk celery, chopped
- 1 bunch fresh parsley, chopped
- 1 yellow onion, chopped
- 1 tablespoon light Miso paste

For the Filling:
- 1 tablespoon extra-virgin olive oil
- ¾ cup diced red onion
- 1 clove garlic, minced
- ½ pound fresh mushrooms, sliced
- 1 cup kale, chopped
- 1 (12 oz) package of firm tofu, crumbled
- 1 tablespoon nutritional yeast
- 1 teaspoon paprika

For the Gravy:
- 2 tablespoons olive oil
- 1/8 cup whole wheat flour
- 2 teaspoons nutritional yeast
- 1 tablespoon Miso broth

DIRECTIONS

1. Whenever you crumble firm tofu into a casserole dish like this, combined with spices or sauces of any kind, you end up with a creamy texture that is reminiscent of ricotta or feta cheese. This is a great way to bring Sirtfoods into a recipe without losing the richness that you crave.
2. Preheat oven to 400 degrees F.
3. Peel and quarter potatoes. Place in a medium or large size pot with water to cover. Add garlic, celery, parsley, and yellow onion. Bring to a boil, cover, and simmer over medium-low heat for 15 to 20 minutes or until potatoes are very tender.
4. To Make Filling: While potatoes are cooking, heat 1 tablespoon oil in a large skillet and sauté onion and garlic over medium heat for 1 minutes, then add mushrooms and kale and sauté for 2 additional minutes.
5. Crumble tofu in chunks into the skillet and sauté briefly, mixing well. Stir in, yeast, thyme and paprika. Mix well and sauté, stirring frequently, for 20 minutes over medium heat.
6. To Make Potato Crust: When they are cooked, transfer potatoes from water to a large bowl, reserving 3 ½ cups of the remaining stock. Whisk the miso paste and oil, to 1 cup of the potato stock and add to the potatoes a little at a time, mashing potatoes as you add the stock. Add only enough water to moisten potatoes adequately.

7. **Assemble Casserole:** Spoon filling into an oiled, shallow ovenproof casserole dish. Pat down with back of a large spoon.
8. Spread potato crust evenly over filling, smoothing top with a spoon or spatula. Dust evenly with paprika.
9. Bake for 30 to 40 minutes, or until crust is golden
10. **To Make the Gravy:** While casserole bakes, heat oil in a large frying pan. Add flour and yeast, stir with a whisk over medium heat to form a paste. Slowly stir in remaining 2 ½ cups of reserved potato water, whisking as you stir to allow gravy to thicken. Stir in instant miso paste and continue whisking until gravy is thick and smooth; add additional potato water, if necessary.
11. Serve casserole inverted, with crust on the bottom and filling on top. Spoon gravy over top

NUTRITION: Calories: 210 kcal Total Fat: 8 g Saturated Fat: 3.5 g Cholesterol: 15 mg Sodium: 290 mg Total Carbs: 28 g Fiber: 3 g Sugar: 2 g Protein: 7 g

Harvest Nut Roast

Preparation Time: 10 minutes

Cooking Time: 1 hour to 1 and ½ hour

Servings: 4

INGREDIENTS

- ½ cup celery, chopped
- 2 red onions, chopped
- ¾ cup walnuts
- ¾ cup pecan or sunflower meal
- 2 ½ cups soy milk
- 1 teaspoon dried basil
- 1 teaspoon dried lovage
- 3 cups breadcrumbs
- Salt and pepper to taste

DIRECTIONS

1. If you are a fan of meatloaf, you will love this nutty alternative. It is hearty and filling, packed with earthy flavor and satisfying in a way only nuts seem to offer.
2. Preheat oven to 350 degrees F and lightly oil a loaf pan.
3. In a medium size skillet, sauté the chopped celery and onion in 3 teaspoons water until cooked.

4. In a large mixing bowl combine the celery and onion with walnuts, pecan or sunflower meal, soymilk, basil, lovage, breadcrumbs, and salt and pepper to taste; mix well.
5. Place mixture in the prepared loaf pan.
6. Bake for 60 to 90 minutes; until the loaf is cooked through.

NUTRITION: Calories: 592.4 kcal Total Fat: 34.4 g Saturated Fat: 5.5 g Cholesterol: 0 mg Sodium: 37.9 mg Total Carbs: 60.7 g Fiber: 10.7 g Sugar: 4.6 g Protein: 19 g

Sweet Potato and Apple Breakfast Skillet

Preparation Time: 10 minutes

Cooking Time: 20 minutes

Servings: 4

INGREDIENTS

- Extra virgin olive oil – 1 tablespoon
- Apple, diced – 1
- Garlic, minced – 2 cloves
- Red onion, diced – 1
- Sweet potato, peeled and diced – 1
- Black pepper, ground – .25 teaspoon
- Kale, chopped – 2 cups
- Chicken apple sausage, sliced – 4 links
- Sea salt – .5 teaspoon

DIRECTIONS

1. You can use whatever your favorite variety and brand of chicken apple sausage is, but I prefer the Aidells brand. There are even vegetarian options for the sausage, such as the one by Field Roast. Another option is that while you can serve this hash plain, you can also top it off with a fried egg, if you would like.

2. Pour the olive oil into a large cast iron skillet and allow it to warm over medium heat. Add in the sweet potatoes and onion, cooking until tender, about seven minutes.
3. Add the sliced sausage and apple into the skillet, allowing it to cook for five additional minutes, being sure to stir occasionally.
4. Stir in the kale and seasonings, allowing it to cook for a couple more minutes, just until the kale has wilted. Remove the sweet potato skillet from the heat and serve alone or with eggs.

NUTRITION: Calories: 115.3 kcal Total Fat: 5 g Saturated Fat: 1.5 g Cholesterol: 46.5 mg Sodium: 34.3 mg Total Carbs: 15.9 g Fiber: 2.1 g Sugar: 8.8 g Protein: 3.1 g

Cinnamon Apple Quinoa

Preparation Time: 10 minutes

Cooking Time: 15 minutes

Servings: 2

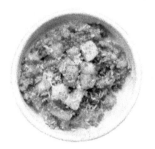

INGREDIENTS

- Quinoa - .5 cup
- Water – 1.5 cups
- Apples, peeled and diced – 2
- Cinnamon – 2 teaspoons
- Sea salt - .25 teaspoon
- Honey – 2 tablespoons

DIRECTIONS

1. By cooking the apples and the quinoa together, you are infusing the quinoa with their sweet flavor. This is further complemented by sweet honey (ideally local raw honey) and cinnamon. This dish is a great option to make in advance, as it reheats well.
2. Add the apples, quinoa, sea salt, and water to a saucepan. Bring the water, apples, and quinoa to a boil before reducing the heat to low, covering the quinoa mixture with a lid, and allowing it to simmer for about twenty minutes. It is ready when the water has been absorbed by the quinoa and the apples are tender.

3. Stir in the cinnamon and divide the quinoa between two serving dishes. Drizzle the honey over the top before enjoying.

NUTRITION: Calories: 229.3 kcal Total Fat: 3.2 g Saturated Fat: 0 g Cholesterol: 0 mg Sodium: 35.5 mg Total Carbs: 35.6 g Fiber: 3.3 g Sugar: 4.2 g Protein: 6.1 g

Turkey Mole Tacos

Preparation Time: 10 minutes

Cooking Time: 15 minutes

Servings: 3

INGREDIENTS

- Lean ground turkey - .75 pound
- Green onion, chopped – 4 stalks
- Garlic cloves, minced – 2
- Celery, chopped – 1 rib
- Roasted sweet peppers, chopped, and drained – 3.5 ounces
- Diced tomatoes, canned – 7 ounces
- Corn tortillas, 6 inches, warmed – 6
- Red onion, thinly sliced – 1
- Walnuts, roasted, chopped – 2 tablespoons
- Dark chocolate, chopped – 2 ounces
- Sea salt - .25 teaspoon
- Chili powder – 4 teaspoons
- Cumin - .5 teaspoon
- Cinnamon, ground - .125 teaspoon

DIRECTIONS

1. These tacos have a rich and deep flavor thanks to the mole, which is then complemented by the fresh red onion. The

meat is easily stored in the freezer until you plan to enjoy and assemble the tacos.

2. In a large skillet that is non-stick cook the ground turkey with the green onions, celery, and garlic over medium heat. Cook until there is no pink remaining, the turkey has reached a temperature of one-hundred and sixty-five degrees, and the vegetables are tender.
3. Into the skillet with the cooked turkey add the canned tomatoes, roasted red peppers, cinnamon, chocolate, chili powder, cumin, and sea salt. Allow the liquid from the tomatoes to come to a boil before reducing the heat to medium-low, covering the skillet with a lid, and simmering for ten minutes. Stir occasionally to prevent sticking and burning.
4. Remove the cooked ground turkey from the heat and stir in the walnuts.
5. Divide the taco meat between the corn tortillas, topping it off with the sliced red onion. Serve while warm.

NUTRITION: Calories: 369 kcal Total Fat: 15 g Saturated Fat: 0 g Cholesterol: 75 mg Sodium: 612 mg Total Carbs: 37 g Fiber: 6 g Sugar: 0 g Protein: 22 g

Sweet and Sour Tofu

Preparation Time: 10 minutes

Cooking Time: 15 minutes

Servings: 4

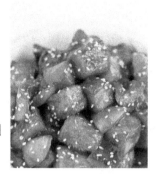

INGREDIENTS
- Tofu, firm – 14 ounces
- Cornstarch – 8 tablespoons, divid
- Egg white – 1
- Pineapple, chopped – 1 cup
- Bell pepper, chopped – 2
- Rice vinegar – 6 tablespoons
- Date sugar – 6 tablespoons
- Tamari sauce – 2 tablespoons
- Sea salt – 1 teaspoon
- Tomato paste – 2 tablespoons
- Water – 2 teaspoons
- Cornstarch – 2 tablespoons
- Sesame seeds, toasted – 1 teaspoon

DIRECTIONS
1. This is a delicious and easy sweet and sour tofu, which you can serve over vegetables such as sautéed cauliflower and kale or grains such as buckwheat or fried rice. Whatever you choose to serve it with, you are sure to love this entree. While this recipe calls for an egg white, you can replace it with three to four tablespoons of aquafaba.
2. Line an aluminum baking sheet with kitchen parchment or a silicone sheet and set the oven to Fahrenheit three-hundred and fifty degrees.

3. Begin by pressing your tofu and then slicing it into bite-sized cubes. Sprinkle two of the eight divided tablespoons of cornstarch over the tofu, tossing it until the tofu is evenly coated.
4. Place the remaining six tablespoons of divided cornstarch in one bowl and the egg white (or aquafaba) in another.
5. Dip a few tofu cubes at a time first in the egg white and then in the cornstarch. Transfer the breaded cubes to the prepared baking sheet and continue the process until all the cubes are prepared. Arrange the tofu cubes on the pan evenly so that they do not touch, and then bake until crispy, about fifteen to twenty minutes.
6. While the tofu cooks, whisk together the rice vinegar, date sugar, tamari sauce, sea salt, tomato paste, water, two tablespoons of corn starch, and the sesame seeds.
7. Add the peppers and pineapple to a large skillet and sauté them until slightly tender. Add in the mixed sauce and deglaze the skillet. Add the cooked tofu to the skillet and continue to cook it in the sauce until it is coated and sticky and the sauce has thickened.
8. Serve while warm over brown rice or buckwheat.

NUTRITION: Calories: 207.2 kcal Total Fat: 11.7 g Saturated Fat: 2.6 g Cholesterol: 5.2 mg Sodium: 40.1 mg Total Carbs: 12.7 g Fiber: 3.5 g Sugar: 3.3 g Protein: 18.1 g

Tofu Tikka Masala

Preparation Time: 15 minutes

Cooking Time: 20 minutes

Servings: 4

INGREDIENTS

- Tofu, extra-firm, sliced into bite-sized cubes – 14 ounces
- Cumin – 1 teaspoon
- Ginger, peeled and grated – 2 teaspoons
- Sweet paprika - .5 teaspoon
- Turmeric - .5 teaspoon
- Garlic, minced – 2 cloves
- Garam masala – 1.5 teaspoons
- Coriander powder - .5 teaspoon
- Cayenne - .25 teaspoon
- Tomato passata (if not available use puree) – 1 cup
- Coconut milk, full-fat – 14 ounces
- Olive oil – 2 tablespoons
- Red onion, diced – 1
- Sea salt – 1 teaspoon

DIRECTIONS

1. Many spices have long been known to have medicinal properties, partly due to their sirtuin contents. This recipe makes use of many types of these spices, as well as tofu and

red onion, to increase your sirtfood consumption and overall wellbeing.

2. Add the olive oil, red onion, and salt to a skillet and allow it to cook over medium until the onions have become soft, about five minutes. Add in the grated ginger and minced garlic, cooking for a minute before adding in all the spices. Cook for an additional two minutes, until the spices are fragrant. Keep a close eye on the spices, stirring constantly to avoid burning.

3. Stir the tomato passata or puree into the skillet and allow it to continue cooking until thickened and reduced, about ten to fifteen minutes.

4. Add the tofu and canned coconut milk to the skillet and bring the pan to a boil. Reduce the stove to low and allow the tikka masala to simmer for ten minutes. Serve warm over brown rice or buckwheat.

NUTRITION: Calories: 440 kcal Total Fat: 29 g Saturated Fat: 15 g Cholesterol: 0 mg Sodium: 233 mg Total Carbs: 18 g Fiber: 3 g Sugar: 7 g Protein: 24 g

Quick Spaghetti Sauce

Preparation Time: 5 minutes

Cooking Time: 30 minutes

Servings: 4

INGREDIENTS

- 1 (29 ounce) can tomato sauce
- 1 cup mushrooms, chopped
- ½ cup chopped celery
- ¼ cup diced red onion
- ¼ cup Medjool dates, chopped
- ¼ cup walnuts, chopped
- 1 tomato, quartered
- 1 large orange, quartered
- 1 tablespoon garlic, minced

DIRECTIONS

1. Homemade tomato sauce is incredibly simple to make simply by boiling, peeling and pureeing tomatoes. However, unless you reduce it, the result is considerably waterier than a canned variety. When you are shopping, remember to look at the ingredients to make sure the tomato sauce is pure, without any added sugar or salt. Either way, the addition of a little orange will bring an absolutely delightful look of surprise to the face of anyone tasting your sauce.

2. In a large, heavy saucepan combine tomato sauce, mushrooms, celery, red onion, dates, walnuts, tomato, orange, and garlic. Cook on medium-high until vegetables are tender, about 30 minutes.
3. Serve with pasta or vegetable noodle alternative.

NUTRITION: Calories: 90 kcal Total Fat: 2.4 g Saturated Fat: 0 g Sodium: 550 mg Total Carbs: 13.1 g Fiber: 2 g Protein: 2 g

Shepherd's Pie [Vegan]

Preparation Time: 25 minutes

Cooking Time: 1 hour and 10 minutes

Servings: 4

INGREDIENTS

For the mashed potatoes:
- 6 large potatoes, peeled and cubed
- ½ cup soymilk
- ¼ cup extra virgin olive oil
- 2 teaspoons salt

For the bottom layer:
- 1 tablespoon extra-virgin olive oil
- 1 yellow onion, chopped
- 3 carrots, chopped
- 3 stalks celery, chopped
- ½ cup frozen peas
- 1 tomato, chopped
- 1 teaspoon dried parsley
- 1 teaspoon dried lovage
- 1 teaspoon dried oregano
- 3 cloves garlic, minced
- 1/2 cup kasha (toasted buckwheat groats)
- 2/3 cup bulgur
- 2 cups fresh mushrooms, diced

DIRECTIONS

1. If you do not announce the vegan-friendly nature of this dish, your taste-testers probably will not even notice there is no actual meat in it. The spiced buckwheat groats, bulgur and diced mushrooms perfectly mimic the ground meat that is usually found in Shepherd's Pie, but with much more sirtuin-activating goodness.
2. Preheat oven to 350 degrees F and spray a 2-quart baking dish with cooking spray.
3. Place the potatoes into a large pot with enough cold water to cover them completely. Bring the water to a boil and then reduce heat to a low boil until the potatoes until tender, about 20 minutes. Drain and transfer to a large bowl.
4. Using a hand blender, mix the soymilk, olive oil, and salt into the potatoes, and blend until smooth. Cover and set aside until your bottom layer are ready.
5. At the same time, in a saucepan, bring 1 ½ cups water with ½ teaspoon salt to a boil. Stir in kasha. Reduce heat and simmer uncovered, for 15 minutes.
6. Add 1 ½ cups more water and bring back to a boil. Add bulgur, cover, and remove from heat. Let stand for 10 minutes.
7. Warm the olive oil in a large pan, and sauté the onion, carrots, celery, frozen peas, and tomato on medium heat

until they start to soften, about 5 minutes. Add mushrooms and cook for another 3 – 4 minutes.

8. Sprinkle flour over vegetables; stir constantly for 2 minutes or until flour starts to brown. Pour remaining 1 ½ cups milk over the vegetables and increase heat to high. Stir until sauce is smooth. Reduce heat and simmer for 5 minutes. Stir in parsley, lovage, oregano, garlic, and salt and pepper to taste.
9. Combine vegetable mixture and kasha mixture in a large bowl and mix well.
10. Spoon into a greased 10" pie pan, and smooth with a spatula. Spread mashed potatoes over top, leaving an uneven surface.
11. Bake until the potatoes turn golden and the Shepherd's Pie is hot throughout, about 30 minutes.

NUTRITION: Calories: 194.3 kcal Total Fat: 2.7 g Saturated Fat: 0.4 g Cholesterol: 0 mg Sodium: 179 mg Total Carbs: 39 g Fiber: 8.3 g Sugar: 4.8 g Protein: 9 g

Spinach and Turkey Lasagna

Preparation Time: 30 minutes

Cooking Time: 25 minutes

Servings: 4

INGREDIENTS
- 9 whole-wheat lasagna noodles
- 1 teaspoon extra virgin olive oil
- ½ cup red onion, chopped
- 1-pound ground turkey breast
- 3 cups tomato sauce
- 1/2 cup mushrooms, sliced
- 1 teaspoon dried parsley
- 1 teaspoon dried lovage
- 1 teaspoon dried oregano
- ¼ teaspoon garlic powder
- Salt and pepper to taste
- 6 cups fresh spinach, chopped
- 2 cups ricotta cheese
- ¼ teaspoon ground nutmeg
- 2 cups shredded mozzarella cheese

DIRECTIONS

1. If you are trying to cut back on your dairy intake or if you simply find lasagna a bit too rich and cheesy for your preferences, try swapping the ricotta cheese for crumbled firm or medium firm tofu. You will be adding another Sirtfood to the dish and it is much lighter, though

surprisingly similar in taste and texture when covered with the sauce.
2. Preheat an oven to 375 degrees F.
3. Bring a large pot of lightly salted water to a boil. Cook lasagna noodles until al dente, approximately 8 minutes. Drain noodles and rinse under cold water.
4. Heat the olive oil in a skillet over medium heat. Stir in the onion and cook until it softens and turns translucent, about 2 minutes.
5. Add ground turkey and cook 5 to 7 minutes more, stirring to break up any large chunks of meat.
6. Stir in tomato sauce, mushrooms, parsley, lovage, oregano, black pepper, and garlic powder. Simmer for 2 minutes and season to taste.
7. Combine spinach, ricotta, and nutmeg in a large bowl.
8. To assemble, arrange 3 noodles lengthwise in the bottom of a greased 9x13 inch baking dish. Spread with 1/3 the spinach-ricotta mixture, 1/3 of the turkey mixture, and 1/3 of the mozzarella. Repeat layers, ending with remaining mozzarella.
9. Bake in preheated oven for 25 minutes. Cool for 5 minutes before serving.

NUTRITION: Calories: 286.2 kcal Total Fat: 9.6 g Saturated Fat: 4.5 g Cholesterol: 62.1 mg Sodium: 547.3 mg Total Carbs: 31.5 g Fiber: 4.9 g Sugar: 4.1 g Protein: 23.4 g

Thai Curry with Chicken and Peanuts

Preparation Time: 20 minutes

Cooking Time: 20 minutes

Servings: 4

INGREDIENTS

- 2 Bird's Eye chili peppers
- 2 tablespoons ginger root, chopped
- 1 tablespoon fresh turmeric root, chopped
- ½ teaspoon cumin
- ½ teaspoon dried coriander
- 1/2 teaspoon ground nutmeg
- 2 tablespoons lemongrass, thinly sliced
- 1 shallot, chopped
- 2 cloves garlic, chopped
- 2 teaspoons fermented shrimp paste
- 2 tablespoons fish sauce
- 3 tablespoons brown sugar
- 2/3-pound skinless, boneless chicken breast, cut into cubes
- 2 tablespoons extra virgin olive oil
- ½ cup roasted peanuts

DIRECTIONS

1. The mere scent of this dish will have your entire neighborhood clambering for a bowl of the heavenly curry.

2. Place the chili peppers in a bowl; pour enough water over the chili peppers to cover. Allow the peppers to soak until softened, about 10 minutes. Drain, chop the peppers finely and set aside.
3. In a large bowl, add the ginger and turmeric root, cumin, coriander, lemongrass, shallot, garlic, shrimp paste, and chopped chili peppers and mash into a paste. Stir the fish sauce and sugar into the paste.
4. Add the chicken to the paste and toss to coat the evenly.
5. Cover bowl and marinate for at least 20 minutes or up to 24 hours in the refrigerator.
6. Heat the oil in a large skillet over medium heat and cook the chicken until no longer pink in the center and the juices run clear, 5 to 7 minutes.
7. Stir 2 cups of water into the pan and add the peanuts.
8. Bring to a simmer and cook until thickened, 20 to 30 minutes. You can also cook this at a lower temperature for up to 2 hours.

NUTRITION: Calories: 496 kcal Total Fat: 35.13 g Saturated Fat: 17.897 g Cholesterol: 108 mg Sodium: 221 mg Total Carbs: 12.16 g Fiber: 4.7 g Sugar: 4.68 g Protein: 35.95 g

Red Lentil Curry

Preparation Time: 10 minutes

Cooking Time: 20 minutes

Servings: 4

INGREDIENTS

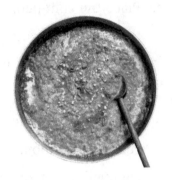

- 2 cups whole red lentils
- 1 large red onion, diced
- 1 tablespoon extra-virgin olive oil
- 1 ½ tablespoons curry paste
- 2 tablespoons curry powder
- 1 teaspoon chili powder
- 1 teaspoon ground turmeric
- 1 teaspoon ground cumin
- 1 teaspoon salt
- 1 teaspoon sugar
- 3 cloves garlic, minced
- 1" section of fresh ginger root, peeled and minced
- 1 (14.25 ounce) can crushed tomatoes

DIRECTIONS

1. Lentils and curry are a match made in heaven. The soft and creamy legumes soak up the curry sauce and ideal for pouring over rice or scooping up with fresh naan.

2. Rinse the lentils in a fine mesh sieve under cold water until the water runs clear - this will prevent your lentils from getting gummy.
3. Transfer the lentils to a medium-sized pot with enough water to cover completely and simmer covered until they are just starting to become tender, about 15 – 20 minutes. Add additional water, as necessary.
4. In the meantime, warm the oil in a large skillet and sauté the onions until they are golden.
5. In a separate bowl, combine the curry paste, curry powder, chili powder, turmeric, cumin, salt, sugar, garlic, and ginger and mix well.
6. When the onions are translucent, add the curry mixture and cook on high, stirring constantly for 2 - 3 minutes.
7. Add in the crushed tomato and reduce the heat. Let the curry blend simmer until the lentils are ready.
8. When the lentils are cooked to your liking, drain well, and add to the curry sauce, mixing well.
9. Serve immediately.

NUTRITION: Calories: 271.6 kcal Total Fat: 2.4 g Saturated Fat: 0.2 g Cholesterol: 0 mg Sodium: 5.8 mg Total Carbs: 53.9 g Fiber: 4.8 g Sugar: 0 g Protein: 8.4 g

Spiced Fish Tacos with Fresh Corn Salsa

Preparation Time: 10 minutes

Cooking Time: 20 minutes

Servings: 4

INGREDIENTS

- 1 cup corn
- 1/2 cup red onion, diced
- 1 cup jicama, peeled and chopped
- 1/2 cup red bell pepper, diced
- 1 cup fresh cilantro leaves, finely chopped
- 1 lime, zested and juiced
- 2 tablespoons sour cream
- 2 tablespoons cayenne pepper
- Salt and pepper to taste
- 8 (4 ounce) fillets tilapia
- 2 tablespoons olive oil
- 8 corn tortillas, warmed

DIRECTIONS

1. If you do not have any available, you can substitute for water chestnuts, celery, or radishes.
2. Preheat grill for high heat.

3. For the Corn Salsa: In a medium bowl, mix together corn, red onion, jicama, red bell pepper, and cilantro. Stir in lime juice and zest.
4. Brush each fillet with olive oil, and sprinkle with the cayenne and season to taste.
5. Arrange fillets on grill and cook for 3 minutes per side. For each fish taco, top two corn tortillas with fish, sour cream, and corn salsa.

NUTRITION: Calories: 297.1 kcal Total Fat: 10.1 g Saturated Fat: 1.4 g Cholesterol: 34.9 mg Sodium: 79.6 mg Total Carbs: 28.2 g Fiber: 6.3 g Sugar: 8.3 g Protein: 25.9 g

Conclusion

Resveratrol shot to popularity in 2003 when a research facility of researchers run by David Sinclair found that this compound, found most normally in the skins of red grapes, copied the impacts of calorie limitation and actuated sirtuins that drawn out the life of cells. Subsequently the 'red wine encourages you live more' way of thinking that is become progressively mainstream bandied about at the bar.

Be that as it may, Hirschey brings up, 'most of studies have been done utilizing test frameworks in the lab, generally on mice or natural product flies, or legitimately into cells. To get resveratrol's enemy of maturing impacts from red wine, you'd need to drink up to 40 liters every day.' Which makes you wonder how much kale you should pack so as to get thinner?

The nutraceutical business is as of now one stage ahead, with resveratrol supplements effectively accessible.

Actually, you do not need to, particularly not to begin. Currently, we are adapted to be snappy and proficient, and to be brisk we have been acquainted with inexpensive food and handled nourishment.

I think what many individuals foul up as do I (during the time spent fixing my diet) is to think about the nourishment being removed, so obviously with that sort of reasoning it turns out to be almost difficult to go for a superfood/raw food diet. Be that as it may, if we have a go at including the superfood/raw food into our current diet, things like crude vegetables, sprouts, natural products, and juices, you will not experience considerable difficulties exchanging. In the wake of adding these natural products to your diet you may not be as eager and when you are not ravenous, you will not surrender to purchasing inexpensive food and prepared nourishment.

Since you will have more opportunity to consider your buys and you have gotten increasingly acclimated with eating more advantageous. If you need that steak or even a McDonald's cheeseburger, you can get yourself it, and it will taste so much better... or on the other hand you might be fortunate to the point that you won't need it by any stretch of the imagination. When you begin eating Superfoods however, you will begin to see how great you feel and the amount more vitality you have, that cheeseburger just will not look as great to you any longer.

During the time spent changing your diet and after changing you would like no doubt however, that you are getting enough of the correct sorts of sustenance. Eating Superfoods/crude nourishments is not simply enough you have to do some exploration on the most proficient method to add your fundamental proteins to your new diet. Recall before you got your protein through your meat yet now you need to get it through your vegetables and crude nourishment, so you have to recognize what to eat and what blends you have to eat to get enough proteins.

One approach to do this is to present another vegetable or crude dish each week. By doing this you will adjust to the new tastes and surfaces and you will begin feeling more regrettable and more terrible for each time you go for inexpensive food or handled nourishment. I hope you enjoyed reading and good luck on your sirtfood diet journey!

Sirtfood Diet Cookbook

The Complete and Easy Recipe Book to Activate Your Skinny Gene, Lose Weight Fast, and Burn Fat with Weekly Meal Plans

Molly Ross

Introduction

Obesity is slowly becoming one of the most serious issues that occurred in Western societies. It is usually favored by lack of activity, even stress, but we can all agree that the food we eat is making us quickly gain weight. Perhaps you are struggling to lose some weight. Perhaps you have an active lifestyle with frequent visits to the gym but still not having the results you expect. This is because you are making some huge mistakes when it comes to your nutrition and/or your workout is not intense enough.

In most of the cases, the nutrition is to blame because we stuff ourselves with plenty of high-calorie and low-nutrient foods. I think we can all agree that the kinds of food consumed a few centuries ago had a better quality than the ones we eat today. Everything was a lot more natural back then, and you didn't have to eat massive amounts to get satisfied. The big issue is with processed food, as it takes the nutrients out of food for the sake of profits. Chemicals are used to "alter" the quality of food, and they are going straight into our bodies. No wonder why we are becoming so fat all of a sudden. The processed food we eat can be compared to the concentrated food of farm animals. It is designed to make us addicted and to make us fat. This is the sad truth!

Yes, I'm afraid that processed food causes addiction. There are too many people addicted to fast foods, snacks, doughnuts, and sodas full of sugar. You can be shocked at the number of calories you consume each day. People often have the wrong impression that more calories mean more energy! Well, yeah! But only if you burn them, not consume them! That's right! Physical exercise can give you energy, not the number of calories you eat. Overeating will make you sleepy instead of feeling more energized.

If we analyze our standard diet, we can easily conclude that we mostly eat carbs. This is what causes most of our nutrition-related issues. Calorie restriction is one antidote for this problem. Others have tried fasting correlated with an LCHF (low-carb, high-fat) diet, or even more radical diets. Unless you stick to a healthy diet and let it become your feeding habit, there's no way you can succeed. There are too many people who can't stick to diets, and they start to gain the weight they lost (with the help of a radical diet) by turning back to their old eating habits.

This book is suggesting a slightly different approach, the food diet. You are probably not even knowing what this diet is about, or you're very reluctant about it since you are too skeptical about diets in general. It is not magic or a scam; this diet really works. Don't believe me? Well, are you wondering how Adele lost so many pounds lately? By trying this diet! This book will provide extremely important information about sirtuins, how this diet works, and plenty of recipes for a very exciting four-week meal plan. Sounds interesting?

Introduction

The Sirtfood Diet

The sirtfood diet can't be classified as low-carb or low-fat. This diet is quite different from its many precursors while advocating many of the same things: the ingestion of fresh, plant-based foods. As the name implies, this is a sirtuin based diet, but what are sirtuins and why have you never heard about them before?

There are seven sirtuin proteins – SIRT-1 to SIRT-71. They can be found throughout your cells and the cells of every animal on the planet. Sirtuins are found in almost every living organism and in almost every part of the cell, controlling what goes on. Supplement company Elysium Health, likens the body's cells to an office with sirtuins acting as the CEO, helping the cells react to internal and external changes. They govern what is done, when it's done, and who does is.

Of the seven sirtuins, one works in your cell's cytoplasm, three in the cell's mitochondria, and another three in the cell's nucleus. They have a wide number of jobs to perform, but mostly they remove acetyl groups from other proteins. These acetyl groups signal that the protein they are attached to is available to perform its function. Sirtuins remove the available flag and get the protein ready to use.

Sirtuins sound pretty crucial to your body's normal function, so why is that you've never heard of them before?

The first sirtuin to be discovered was SIR2, a gene discovered in the 1970s which controlled the ability of fruit flies to mate. It wasn't until the 1990s that scientists discovered other, similar proteins, in almost every form of life. Every organism had a different number of sirtuins – bacteria has one and yeast has five. Experiments on mice show they have the same number as humans, seven.

Sirtuins have been shown to prolong life in yeast and in mice. There is, so far, no evidence of the same effect in human beings, however, these sirtuins are present in almost every form of life and many scientists are hopeful that if organisms as far apart as yeast and mice can see the same effect from sirtuin activation, this may also extend to humans.

In addition to sirtuins, our bodies need another substance called noicotineamide adenine dinucleotide for cells to function properly. Elysium (see above) likens this substance to the money a company needs to keep operating. Like any CEO, a sirtuin can only keep the company working properly if the cash flow is sufficient. NAD+ was first discovered in 1906. You get your supply of NAD+ from your diet by eating foods made up the building blocks of NAD+.

Fun Facts about Sirtuins

1. Mice that have been engineered to have high levels of SIRT-1 are both more active and leaner than normal, while mice that lack

SIRT-1 altogether are fatter and more prone to various metabolic conditions.

2. Add the fact that levels of SIRT-1 are much lower in obese people than in those of a "healthy" weight and the case for the importance of sirtuins in weight loss becomes compelling.

3. By making a permanent change to your diet and adding the best sirtfoods to your eating plan, the authors of the sirtfood diet believe everyone can achieve better health, all without losing muscle mass.

To Sum Up

Exercise and calorie restriction are both sources of stress which encourage our bodies to adapt to changing circumstances. If the stress becomes too great the result can be injury, the body can even die, but at lower levels, we adapt and this temporary, low-level stress is key to many physiological changes.

For example, stress on muscles, enough but not too much, is what makes the body increase muscle mass.

Similarly, the authors of the sirtfood diet found that it is when the body is stressed, by exercise or low-calorie intake, that the effect of sirtuins kicks in and it is this effect that can be reproduced by a diet rich in SIRT foods.

The Discovery and History of Sirtuins

There were different quantities of sirtuins in every creature. For instance, yeast has five sirtuins, microscopic organisms have one, mice have seven, and people have seven.

The way that sirtuins were found across species implies they were "saved" with development. Qualities that are "rationed" have all-inclusive capacities in numerous or all species. What was at this point to be known, however, was the means by which significant sirtuins would end up being.

In 1991, Elysium fellow benefactor and MIT scholar Leonard Guarente, nearby alumni understudies Nick Austriaco and Brian Kennedy, led trials to all the more likely see how yeast matured. By some coincidence, Austriaco attempted to develop societies of different yeast strains from tests he had put away in his ice chest for quite a long time, which made a distressing domain for the strains. Just a portion of these strains could develop from here, yet Guarente and his group identified an example: The strains of yeast that endure the best in the cooler were likewise the longest lived. This gave direction to Guarente so he could concentrate exclusively on these long-living strains of yeast.

This prompted the identification of SIR2 as a quality that advanced life span in yeast. It's critical to note more research is required on SIR2's belongings in people. The Guarente lab consequently found that expelling SIR2 abbreviated yeast life range significantly, while in particular, expanding the quantity of duplicates of the SIR2 quality from one to two expanded the life length in yeast. In any case, what initiated SIR2 normally presently couldn't seem to be found.

This is the place acetyl bunches become possibly the most important factor. It was at first idea that SIR2 may be a deacetylating protein — which means it expelled those acetyl gatherings — from different atoms, yet nobody knew if this were valid since all endeavors to show this movement in a test tube demonstrated negative. Guarente and his group had the option to find that SIR2 in yeast could just deacetylate different proteins within the sight of the coenzyme NAD+, nicotinamide adenine dinucleotide.

In Guarente's own words: "Without NAD+, SIR2 sits idle. That was the basic finding on the circular segment of sirtuin science."

Benefits of Sirtfoods

Top 20 Sirtfoods

- Turmeric
- Birds-eye chillies
- Capers
- Celery
- Coffee
- Extra virgin olive oil
- Green tea
- Kale
- Walnuts
- Lovage
- Medjool dates
- Buckwheat
- Parsley
- Red chicory
- Red wine
- Rocket
- Chocolate
- Cocoa
- Strawberries

Appetite for Fasting

That takes us to fast. Consistently, the lifelong restriction of food intake has been shown to extend the life expectancy of lower organisms and mammals. This extraordinary finding is the reason for the custom of caloric restriction among some individuals, where daily calorie consumption is lowered by about 20 to 30 percent, as well as its popularized offshoot, intermittent fasting, which has become a standard weight-loss method, made famous by the likes of the 5:2 diet, or Fast Method. While we're still looking for proof of improved survival for humans from these activities, there's confirmation of benefits for what we might term "health span"— chronic disease decreases, and fat starts to melt away.

But let's be real, no matter how significant the benefits, fasting week in, week out, is a grueling enterprise that most of us don't want to sign up for. Even if we do, most of us are not able to stick to this.

Besides this, there are risks to fasting, mainly if we practice it for a long time. We mentioned in the introduction the side effects of hunger, irritability, fatigue, muscle loss and slowdown in metabolism. Yet current fasting programs could also place us at risk of starvation, impacting our well-being due to a decreased intake of essential nutrients. Fasting systems are also entirely inappropriate for large proportions of the populace, such as infants, women during breastfeeding, and very likely older adults.

Although fasting has clearly proven advantages, it's not the magic bullet we'd like it to be. It had to wonder, is this really the way God was meant to make us slim and healthy? There's certainly a better path out there.

Our breakthrough came when we discovered that our ancient sirtuin genes were activated by mediating the profound benefits of caloric restriction and fasting. It may be helpful to think of sirtuins as guards at the crossroads of energy status and survival to better understand this. There, what they do is react to pressures. If nutrition is in short supply, there is a rise in tension on our cells, just as we see in the caloric restriction. The sirtuins sensed this, which then switched on and transmitted a constellation of powerful signals that radically altered the behavior of cells.

An Energy for Exercise

It's not just caloric restriction and fasting that activates sirtuins; exercise does too. Sirtuins orchestrate the profound benefits of exercise just as they do in fasting. Yet while we are urged to participate in routine, moderate exercise for its multitude of advantages, it is not the method by which we are expected to focus our efforts on weight-loss. Research shows that the human body has developed ways of adapting spontaneously and reducing the amount of energy that we spend while exercising, seven implying that in order for exercise to be a successful weight-loss strategy, we need to devote considerable time and effort. The grueling fitness plans are the way Nature intended us to maintain a healthy weight is even more questionable in the light of studies now showing that too much activity can be harmful— weakening our immune systems, harming the liver, and leading to an early death.

So far, we have discovered that the key to activating our sirtuin genes is if we want to lose weight and be healthy. Up until now, diet and meditation have been the two proven ways to achieve this.

As we will know early, these are the wonderful foods which are especially rich in specific natural plant chemicals, which have the ability to communicate to our sirtuin genes and turn them on. Essentially, they mimic the results of diet and exercise, which offer impressive advantages by burning fat in doing so., muscle building, and health-boosting that was previously unattainable.

Sirtfood Diet– Phase 1 & Phase 2

The diet is mainly divided into two phases: the first lasts one week and the other lasts 14 days.

Phase 1 (The Most Effective): Three Kilos in Seven Days

It is the "supersonic" phase: the calorie restriction is combined with a diet rich in Sirt foods. The novelty compared to other diets is that it fattens and fattens the muscles. Two different moments. Days 1-3 are the most intense, and during this time you can consume a maximum of one thousand calories per day. You must consume 3 Sirt green juices and a solid meal.

On days 4-7 assigned the intake of one thousand five hundred calories daily. You have to take two green Sirt juices and two solid meals. Phase 1 is the most intense, in which the best results are seen and which allows you to lose up to 3.5 kilos.

The menu to follow includes a "fixed" part, the one relating to green juice created by nutritionists that helps to moderate the appetite of the brain, and one that varies daily.

The green juice recipe is simple and includes all-natural products: 75 g of curly kale, 30 g of arugula and 5 g of parsley must be centrifuged, together with 150 g of green celery with the leaves and 1/2 green apple, grated. Everything must be completed with half a squeezed lemon and half a teaspoon of Matcha tea.

Here is more in detail the program of the first week:

Monday - Wednesday: 3 Sirt green juices to be taken on waking up, mid-morning and mid-afternoon; 1 solid meal of animal or vegan protein (for example, turkey escalope or buckwheat noodles with tofu) accompanied by vegetables, always ending with 15-20 g of 85% dark chocolate.

Thursday - Sunday: 2 Sirt green juices and 2 solid meals, remembering to always vary the main course chosen, from salmon fillet to vegetable tabbouleh to buckwheat spaghetti with celery and kale.

Phase 2 (Maintenance), For 14 Days

Every day, for 14 days, you will eat three balanced meals, chock full of Sirt foods, drink a Sirt green juice and consume 1-2 Sirt snacks. Green juice should be taken in the morning as soon as you wake up or at least 30 minutes before breakfast, or mid-morning. The evening meal must be eaten by 7pm.

Phase 2 is the maintenance phase. During this period the goal is the consolidation of weight loss, although the possibility of losing weight is not excluded. To do all this, just feed on the exceptional food's rich in sirtuins. It lasts 14 days, is less restrictive than the first and provides for sirt foods at will: 3 solid meals plus two juices. The important thing is that they are balanced.

The positive aspects of this diet are:

One is the fact that the calorie limit is indicative and not a goal to be achieved. Another advantage is that the dishes on offer are very satisfying. This way you won't have the hunger attacks typical of other diets. The caloric restriction of the diet even in the most intensive phase is not drastic and Sirt foods have a satiating effect, which prevents us from getting hungry at meals

And then?

As already explained in the introduction, the sirtfood diet cannot (and must not) continue indefinitely and for a very long period of time. Rather, it must be done in cycles, once, two or three times a year. However, the "lifestyle" sirt can continue even after completing the phase.

Sirt foods can be eaten all year round, continuing to speed up the metabolism. However, this should not be combined with a very strong calorie restriction, but only avoid eating unhealthy foods, such as fried, sweet or unsaturated fats. Your persistence will make the difference between success and failure, remember: this is not a shot, but a marathon!

Sirt cycles are simply a boost, a powerful weapon in your arsenal that you can use twice a year (depending on your body of course), but you can have a healthy lifestyle all year round, perhaps combined with a regular physical exercise.

Breakfast Recipes – Phase 1

10. Main Baby Spinach Snack

Preparation time: 10 minutes

Cooking time: 10 minutes

Servings: 3

Ingredients:

- 2 cups baby spinach, washed
- A pinch of black pepper
- ½ tablespoon olive oil
- ½ teaspoon garlic powder

Directions:

1. Spread the baby spinach on a lined baking sheet, add oil, black pepper and garlic powder, toss a bit, introduce in the oven, bake at 350 degrees F for 10 minutes, divide into bowls and serve as a snack.
2. Enjoy!

Nutrition: Calories 125 Fat 4 Fiber 1, Carbs 4 Protein 2

Potato Bites

Preparation time: 10 minutes

Cooking time: 20 minutes

Servings: 3

Ingredients:

- 1 potato, sliced
- 2 bacon slices, already cooked and crumbled
- 1 small avocado, pitted and cubed
- Cooking spray

Directions:

1. Spread potato slices on a lined baking sheet, spray with cooking oil, introduce in the oven at 350 degrees F, bake for 20 minutes, arrange on a platter, top each slice with avocado and crumbled bacon and serve as a snack.
2. Enjoy!

Nutrition: Calories 180 Fat 4 Fiber 1 Carbs 8 Protein 6

Sesame Dip

Preparation time: 10 minutes

Cooking time: 0 minutes

Servings: 6

Ingredients:

- 1 cup sesame seed paste, pure
- Black pepper to the taste
- 1 cup veggie stock
- ½ cup lemon juice
- ½ teaspoon cumin, ground
- 3 garlic cloves, chopped

Directions:

1. In your food processor, mix the sesame paste with black pepper, stock, lemon juice, cumin and garlic, pulse very well, divide into bowls and serve as a party dip.
2. Enjoy!

Nutrition: Calories 120, Fat 12, Fiber 2, Carbs 7, Protein 4

Rosemary Squash Dip

Preparation time: 10 minutes

Cooking time: 40 minutes

Servings: 4

Ingredients:

- 1 cup butternut squash, peeled and cubed
- 1 tablespoon water
- Cooking spray
- 2 tablespoons coconut milk
- 2 teaspoons rosemary, dried
- Black pepper to the taste

Directions:

1. Spread squash cubes on a lined baking sheet, spray some cooking oil, introduce in the oven, bake at 365 degrees F for 40 minutes, transfer to your blender, add water, milk, rosemary and black pepper, pulse well, divide into small bowls and serve
2. Enjoy!

Nutrition: Calories 182 Fat 5 Fiber 7 Carbs 12 Protein 5

Bean Spread

Preparation time: 10 minutes

Cooking time: 7 hours

Servings: 4

Ingredients:

- 1 cup white beans, dried
- 1 teaspoon apple cider vinegar
- 1 cup veggie stock
- 1 tablespoon water

Directions:

1. In your slow cooker, mix beans with stock, stir, cover, cook on Low for 6 hours, drain, transfer to your food processor, add vinegar and water, pulse well, divide into bowls and serve.
2. Enjoy!

Nutrition: Calories 181 Fat 6 Fiber 5 Carbs 9 Protein 7

Eggplant Salsa

Preparation time: 10 minutes

Cooking time: 10 minutes

Servings: 4

Ingredients:

- 1 and ½ cups tomatoes, chopped
- 3 cups eggplant, cubed
- A drizzle of olive oil
- 2 teaspoons capers
- 6 ounces green olives, pitted and sliced
- 4 garlic cloves, minced
- 2 teaspoons balsamic vinegar
- 1 tablespoon basil, chopped
- Black pepper to the taste

Directions:

1. Heat up a pan with the oil over medium-high heat, add eggplant, stir and cook for 5 minutes.
2. Add tomatoes, capers, olives, garlic, vinegar, basil and black pepper, toss, cook for 5 minutes more, divide into small cups and serve cold.
3. Enjoy!

Nutrition: Calories 120 Fat 6 Fiber 5 Carbs 9 Protein 7

Carrots and Cauliflower Spread

Preparation time: 10 minutes

Cooking time: 40 minutes

Servings: 4

Ingredients:

- 1 cup carrots, sliced
- 2 cups cauliflower florets
- ½ cup cashews
- 2 and ½ cups water
- 1 cup almond milk
- 1 teaspoon garlic powder
- ¼ teaspoon smoked paprika

Directions:

1. In a small pot, mix the carrots with cauliflower, cashews and water, stir, cover, bring to a boil over medium heat, cook for 40 minutes, drain and transfer to a blender.
2. Add almond milk, garlic powder and paprika, pulse well, divide into small bowls and serve
3. Enjoy!

Nutrition: Calories 201 Fat 7 Fiber 4 Carbs 7 Protein 7

Italian Veggie Salsa

Preparation time: 10 minutes

Cooking time: 10 minutes

Servings: 4

Ingredients:

- 2 red bell peppers, cut into medium wedges
- 3 zucchinis, sliced
- ½ cup garlic, minced
- 2 tablespoons olive oil
- A pinch of black pepper
- 1 teaspoon Italian seasoning

Directions:

1. Heat up a pan with the oil over medium-high heat, add bell peppers and zucchini, toss and cook for 5 minutes.
2. Add garlic, black pepper and Italian seasoning, toss, cook for 5 minutes more, divide into small cups and serve as a snack.
3. Enjoy!

Nutrition: Calories 132 Fat 3 Fiber 3 Carbs 7 Protein 4

Black Bean Salsa

Preparation time: 10 minutes

Cooking time: 0 minutes

Servings: 6

Ingredients:

- 1 tablespoon coconut aminos
- ½ teaspoon cumin, ground
- 1 cup canned black beans, no-salt-added, drained and rinsed
- 1 cup salsa
- 6 cups romaine lettuce leaves, torn
- ½ cup avocado, peeled, pitted and cubed

Directions:

1. In a bowl, combine the beans with the aminos, cumin, salsa, lettuce and avocado, toss, divide into small bowls and serve as a snack.
2. Enjoy!

Nutrition: Calories 181 Fat 4 Fiber 7 Carbs 14 Protein 7

Corn Spread

Preparation time: 10 minutes

Cooking time: 10 minutes

Servings: 6

Ingredients:

- 30 ounces canned corn, drained
- 2 green onions, chopped
- ½ cup coconut cream
- 1 jalapeno, chopped
- ½ teaspoon chili powder

Directions:

1. In a small pan, combine the corn with green onions, jalapeno and chili powder, stir, bring to a simmer, cook over medium heat for 10 minutes, leave aside to cool down, add coconut cream, stir well, divide into small bowls and serve as a spread.
2. Enjoy!

Nutrition: Calories 192 Fat 5 Fiber 10 Carbs 11 Protein 8

Mushroom Dip

Preparation time: 10 minutes

Cooking time: 20 minutes

Servings: 6

Ingredients:

- 1 cup yellow onion, chopped
- 3 garlic cloves, minced
- 1-pound mushrooms, chopped
- 28 ounces tomato sauce, no-salt-added
- Black pepper to the taste

Directions:

1. Put the onion in a pot, add garlic, mushrooms, black pepper and tomato sauce, stir, cook over medium heat for 20 minutes, leave aside to cool down, divide into small bowls and serve.
2. Enjoy!

Nutrition: Calories 215 Fat 4 Fiber 7 Carbs 3 Protein 7

Salsa Bean Dip

Preparation time: 10 minutes

Cooking time: 20 minutes

Servings: 6

Ingredients:

- ½ cup salsa
- 2 cups canned white beans, no-salt-added, drained and rinsed
- 1 cup low-fat cheddar, shredded
- 2 tablespoons green onions, chopped

Directions:

1. In a small pot, combine the beans with the green onions and salsa, stir, bring to a simmer over medium heat, cook for 20 minutes, add cheese, stir until it melts, take off heat, leave aside to cool down, divide into bowls and serve.
2. Enjoy!

Nutrition: Calories 212 Fat 5 Fiber 6 Carbs 10 Protein 8

Mung Sprouts Salsa

Preparation time: 10 minutes

Cooking time: 0 minutes

Servings: 2

Ingredients:

- 1 red onion, chopped
- 2 cups mung beans, sprouted
- A pinch of red chili powder
- 1 green chili pepper, chopped
- 1 tomato, chopped
- 1 teaspoon chaat masala
- 1 teaspoon lemon juice
- 1 tablespoon coriander, chopped
- Black pepper to the taste

Directions:

1. In a salad bowl, mix onion with mung sprouts, chili pepper, tomato, chili powder, chaat masala, lemon juice, coriander and pepper, toss well, divide into small cups and serve.
2. Enjoy!

Nutrition: Calories 100 Fat 2 Fiber 1 Carbs 3 Protein 6

Mung Beans Snack Salad

Preparation time: 10 minutes

Cooking time: 0 minutes

Servings: 6

Ingredients:

- 2 cups tomatoes, chopped
- 2 cups cucumber, chopped
- 3 cups mixed greens
- 2 cups mung beans, sprouted
- 2 cups clover sprouts
- For the salad dressing:
- 1 tablespoon cumin, ground
- 1 cup dill, chopped
- 4 tablespoons lemon juice
- 1 avocado, pitted, peeled and roughly chopped
- 1 cucumber, roughly chopped

Directions:

1. In a salad bowl, mix tomatoes with 2 cups cucumber, greens, clover and mung sprouts.
2. In your blender, mix cumin with dill, lemon juice, 1 cucumber and avocado, blend really well, add this to your salad, toss well and serve as a snack. Enjoy!

Nutrition: Calories 120 Fat 0 Fiber 2 Carbs 1 Protein 6

Sprouts and Apples Snack Salad

Preparation time: 10 minutes

Cooking time: 0 minutes

Servings: 4

Ingredients:

- 1-pound Brussels sprouts, shredded
- 1 cup walnuts, chopped
- 1 apple, cored and cubed
- 1 red onion, chopped
- For the salad dressing:
- 3 tablespoons red vinegar
- 1 tablespoon mustard
- ½ cup olive oil
- 1 garlic clove, minced
- Black pepper to the taste

Directions:

1. In a salad bowl, mix sprouts with apple, onion and walnuts.
2. In another bowl, mix vinegar with mustard, oil, garlic and pepper, whisk really well, add this to your salad, toss well and serve as a snack.
3. Enjoy!

Nutrition: Calories 120 Fat 2 Fiber 2 Carbs 8 Protein 6

Breakfast Recipes – Phase 1

Main Meals Recipes – Phase 1

Salmon and Capers

Preparation time: 15 minutes

Cooking time: 10 minutes

Servings: 4

Ingredients:

- 75g (3oz) Greek yogurt
- 4 salmon fillets, skin removed
- 4 teaspoons Dijon Mustard
- 1 tablespoon capers, chopped
- 2 teaspoons fresh parsley
- Zest of 1 lemon

Directions:

1. In a bowl, mix together the yogurt, mustard, lemon zest, parsley and capers. Thoroughly coat the salmon in the mixture. Place the salmon under a hot grill (broiler) and cook for 3-4 minutes on each side, or until the fish is cooked. Serve with mashed potatoes and vegetables or a large green leafy salad.

Nutrition: 321 calories per serving

Coconut curry

Preparation time: 10 minutes

Cooking time: 2 minutes

Servings: 4

Ingredients:

- 400g (14oz) tinned chopped tomatoes
- 25g (1oz) fresh coriander (cilantro) chopped
- 3 red onions, finely chopped
- 3 cloves of garlic, crushed
- 2 bird's eye chillies
- ½ teaspoon ground coriander (cilantro)
- ½ teaspoon turmeric
- 400mls (14fl oz.) coconut milk
- 1 tablespoons olive oil
- Juice of 1 lime

Directions:

1. Place the onions, garlic, tomatoes, chillies, lime juice, turmeric, ground coriander (cilantro), chillies and half of the fresh coriander (cilantro) into a blender and blitz until you have a smooth curry paste. Heat the olive oil in a frying pan, add the paste and cook for 2 minutes. Stir in the coconut milk and warm it thoroughly. Stir in the fresh coriander (cilantro). Serve with rice

Nutrition: 322 calories per serving

Tofu Thai Curry

Preparation time: 15 minutes

Cooking time: 15 minutes

Servings: 4

Ingredients:

- 400g (14oz) tofu, diced
- 200g (7oz) sugar snap peas
- 5cm (2 inch) chunk fresh ginger root, peeled and finely chopped
- 2 red onions, chopped
- 2 cloves of garlic, crushed
- 2 bird's eye chillies
- 2 tablespoons tomato puree
- 1 stalk of lemon grass, inner stalks only
- 1 tablespoon fresh coriander (cilantro), chopped
- 1 teaspoon cumin
- 300mls (½ pint) coconut milk
- 200mls (7fl oz.) vegetable stock (broth)
- 1 tablespoon virgin olive oil
- Juice of 1 lime

Directions:

1. Heat the oil in a frying pan, add the onion and cook for 4 minutes. Add in the chillies, cumin, ginger, and garlic and cook for 2 minutes. Add the tomato puree, lemon grass,

sugar-snap peas, lime juice and tofu and cook for 2 minutes. Pour in the stock (broth), coconut milk and coriander (cilantro) and simmer for 5 minutes. Serve with brown rice or buckwheat and a handful of rockets (arugula) leaves on the side.

Nutrition: 270 calories per serving

Turkey Curry

Preparation time: 15 minutes

Cooking time: 25 minutes

Servings: 4

Ingredients:

- 450g (1lb) turkey breasts, chopped
- 100g (3½ oz.) fresh rocket (arugula) leaves
- 5 cloves garlic, chopped
- 3 teaspoons medium curry powder
- 2 teaspoons turmeric powder
- 2 tablespoons fresh coriander (cilantro), finely chopped
- 2 bird's-eye chillies, chopped
- 2 red onions, chopped
- 400mls (14fl oz.) full-fat coconut milk
- 2 tablespoons olive oil

Directions:

1. Heat the olive oil in a saucepan, add the chopped red onions and cook them for around 5 minutes or until soft. Stir in the garlic and the turkey and cook it for 7-8 minutes. Stir in the turmeric, chillies and curry powder then add the coconut milk and coriander (cilantro). Bring it to the boil, reduce the heat and simmer for around 10 minutes. Scatter the rocket (arugula) onto plates and spoon the curry on top. Serve alongside brown rice.

Nutrition: 402 calories per serving

Sirtfood Pizza

Preparation time: 15 minutes

Cooking time: 45 minutes

Servings: 6

Ingredients for the dough:

- 7g dry yeast
- 1 teaspoon brown sugar
- 300ml water
- 200g buckwheat flour
- 200g wheat flour for pasta
- 1 tablespoon of olive oil

Directions:

1. Dissolve dry yeast and sugar in water and leave covered for 15 minutes. Then mix the flours. Add the yeast water and oil and make dough.
2. Preheat oven to 425 °. Then knead the dough well again and form two pizzas, each 30 cm in diameter, with a rolling pin on a floured work surface. Or you can form a thin pizza that fits on a whole baking sheet.
3. Spread the pizza dough on a baking tray lined with baking paper.

Ingredients for the sauce:

- 1/2 red onion, finely chopped

- 1 clove of garlic, finely chopped
- 1 teaspoon of olive oil
- 1 teaspoon oregano, dried
- 2 tablespoons red wine
- 1 can of strained tomatoes (400ml)
- 1 pinch of brown sugar
- 5g basil leaves

Directions:

1. Fry the garlic, onion and sugar with olive oil, add the wine and oregano and cook briefly. Then add the tomatoes and cook on low heat for 30 minutes. Then set aside and add the fresh basil leaves.
2. Pizza topping and baking
3. Spread the desired amount of tomato sauce on the dough - leave the edges as free as possible, do not spread too thickly.
4. Then add the desired ingredients, for example
5. Sliced red onion and grilled eggplant
6. Goat cheese and cherry tomatoes
7. Chicken breast (grilled), red onions and olives
8. Kale, chorizo and red onions
9. Then bake for about 12 minutes and, if desired, sprinkle with rocket, pepper and chili flakes.

Nutrition: 354 Calories

Red Coleslaw

Preparation time: 10 minutes

Cooking time: 0 minutes

Servings: 4

Ingredients:

- 1 2/3 pounds red cabbage
- 2 tablespoons ground caraway seeds
- 1 tablespoon whole grain mustard
- 1 1/4 cups mayonnaise, low fat, low sodium
- Salt and black pepper

Directions:

1. Cut the red cabbage into small slices.
2. Take a large-sized bowl and add all the ingredients alongside cabbage.
3. Mix well, season with salt and pepper.
4. Serve and enjoy!

Nutrition: Calories: 406 Fat: 40.8g Carbohydrates: 10g Protein: 2.2g

Avocado Mayo Medley

Preparation time: 5 minutes

Cooking time: 0 minutes

Servings: 4

Ingredients:

- 1 medium avocado, cut into chunks
- ½ teaspoon ground cayenne pepper
- 2 tablespoons fresh cilantro
- ¼ cup olive oil
- ½ cup mayo, low fat and los sodium

Directions:

1. Take a food processor and add avocado, cayenne pepper, lime juice, salt and cilantro.
2. Mix until smooth.
3. Slowly incorporate olive oil, add 1 tablespoon at a time and keep processing between additions.
4. Store and use as needed!

Nutrition: Calories: 231 Fat: 20g Carbohydrates: 5g Protein: 3g

Amazing Garlic Aioli

Preparation time: 5 minutes

Cooking time: Nil

Servings: 4

Ingredients:

- ½ cup mayonnaise, low fat and low sodium
- 2 garlic cloves, minced
- Juice of 1 lemon
- 1 tablespoon fresh-flat leaf Italian parsley, chopped
- 1 teaspoon chives, chopped
- Salt and pepper to taste

Directions:

1. How To:
2. Add mayonnaise, garlic, parsley, lemon juice, chives and season with salt and pepper.
3. Blend until combined well.
4. Pour into refrigerator and chill for 30 minutes.
5. Serve and use as needed!

Nutrition: Calories: 813 Fat: 88g Carbohydrates: 9g Protein: 2g

Easy Seed Crackers

Preparation time: 10 minutes

Cooking time: 60 minutes

Servings: 4

Ingredients:

- 1 cup boiling water
- 1/3 cup chia seeds
- 1/3 cup sesame seeds
- 1/3 cup pumpkin seeds
- 1/3 cup Flaxseeds
- 1/3 cup sunflower seeds
- 1 tablespoon Psyllium powder
- 1 cup almond flour
- 1 teaspoon salt
- ¼ cup coconut oil, melted

Directions:

1. How To:
2. Pre-heat your oven to 300 degrees F.
3. Line a cookie sheet with parchment paper and keep it on the side.

4. Add listed ingredients (except coconut oil and water) to food processor and pulse until ground.
5. Transfer to a large mixing bowl and pour melted coconut oil and boiling water, mix.
6. Transfer mix to prepared sheet and spread into a thin layer.
7. Cut dough into crackers and bake for 60 minutes.
8. Cool and serve. Enjoy!

Nutrition: Total Carbs: 10.6g Fiber: 3g Protein: 5g Fat: 14.6g

Main Meals Recipes – Phase 1 (Part 2)

Sticky Chicken Watermelon Noodle Salad

Preparation time: 10 minutes

Cooking time: 6 minutes

Servings: 3

Ingredients

- 2 pieces of skinny rice noodles
- 1/2 tbsp. sesame oil
- 2 cups watermelon
- Head of bib lettuce
- Half of a lot of scallions
- Half of a lot of fresh cilantro
- 2 skinless, boneless chicken breasts
- 1/2 tbsp. Chinese five-spice
- 1 tbsp. extra virgin olive oil
- Two tbsp. sweet skillet (I utilized a mixture of maple syrup using a dash of tabasco)
- 1 tbsp. sesame seeds
- A couple of cashews - smashed
- Dressing - could be made daily or 2 until

- 1 tbsp. low-salt soy sauce
- 1 teaspoon sesame oil
- 1 tbsp. peanut butter
- Half of a refreshing red chili
- Half of a couple of chives
- Half of a couple of cilantros
- 1 lime - juiced
- 1 small spoonful of garlic

Directions:

1. In a bowl, then completely substituting the noodles in boiling drinking water. They are going to soon be spread out in 2 minutes.
2. On a big sheet of parchment paper, throw the chicken with pepper, salt and also the five-spice.
3. Twist over the paper, subsequently flatten the chicken using a rolling pin.
4. Place into the large skillet with 1 tbsp. of olive oil, turning 3 or 4 minutes, until well charred and cooked through.
5. Drain the noodles and toss with 1 tbsp. of sesame oil onto a sizable serving dish.
6. Place 50% the noodles into the moderate skillet, stirring frequently until crispy and nice.

7. Remove the watermelon skin, then slice the flesh to inconsistent balls and then move to plate.
8. Wash the lettuces and cut into small wedges and also half of a whole lot of leafy greens and scatter on the dish.
9. Place another 1 / 2 the cilantro pack, the soy sauce, coriander, chives, peanut butter, a dab of water, 1 teaspoon of sesame oil and the lime juice in a bowl, then mix till smooth.
10. Set the chicken back to heat, garnish with all the sweet sauce (or my walnut syrup mixture) and toss with the sesame seeds.
11. Pour the dressing on the salad toss gently with clean fingers until well coated, then add crispy noodles and then smashed cashews.
12. Mix chicken pieces and add them to the salad.

Nutrition: 254 calories

Fruity Curry Chicken Salad

Preparation time: 15 minutes

Cooking time: 0 minutes

Servings: 2

Ingredients:

- 4 skinless, boneless chicken pliers - cooked and diced
- 1 tsp. celery, diced
- 4 green onions, sliced
- 1 golden delicious apple peeled, cored and diced
- 1/3 cup golden raisins
- 1/3 cup seedless green grapes, halved
- 1/2 cup sliced toasted pecans
- 1/8 Teaspoon ground black pepper
- 1/2 tsp. curry powder
- 3/4 cup light mayonnaise

Directions:

1. In a big bowl combine the chicken, onion, celery, apple, celery, celery, pecans, pepper, curry powder, and carrot. Mix altogether. Enjoy!

Nutrition: Per serving: 229 carbohydrates 14 grams total fat 44 milligrams cholesterol

Zuppa Toscana

Preparation time: 25 minutes

Cooking time: 1 hour

Servings: 3

Ingredients

- 1 lb. ground Italian sausage
- 1 1/4 tsp. crushed red pepper flakes
- 4 pieces bacon, cut into ½ inch bits
- 1 big onion, diced
- 1 tbsp. minced garlic
- 5 (13.75 oz.) can chicken broth
- 6 celery, thinly chopped
- 1 cup thick cream
- 1/4 bunch fresh spinach, tough stems removed

Directions:

1. Cook that the Italian sausage and red pepper flakes in a pot on medium-high heat until crumbly, browned, with no longer pink, 10 to 15minutes. Drain and put aside.
2. Cook the bacon at the exact Dutch oven over moderate heat until crispy, about 10 minutes, drain, leaving a couple of

tablespoons of drippings together with all the bacon at the bottom of the toaster. Stir in the garlic and onions cook until onions are tender and translucent, about five minutes.

3. Pour the chicken broth to the pot with the onion and bacon mix; contribute to a boil on high temperature. Add the berries, and boil until fork-tender, about 20 minutes. Reduce heat to moderate and stir in the cream and also the cooked sausage – heat throughout. Mix the lettuce to the soup before serving.

Nutrition: Per month: 554 carbs 32.6 grams fat 45.8 grams carbs 19.8 grams protein

Turmeric Chicken & Kale Salad with Honey-Lime Dressing

Preparation time: 20 minutes

Cooking time: 10 minutes

Servings: 2

Ingredients:

For your poultry

- 1 tsp. ghee or 1 tablespoon coconut oil
- 1/2 moderate brown onion, diced
- 250 300 grams / 9 oz. Chicken mince or pops upward chicken thighs
- 1 large garlic clove, finely-chopped
- 1 tsp. turmeric powder
- Optional 1teaspoon lime zest
- Juice of 1/2 lime
- 1/2 tsp. salt

For your salad

- 6 broccoli 2 or two cups of broccoli florets
- 2 tbsp. pumpkin seeds (pepitas)
- 3 big kale leaves, stalks removed and sliced
- Optional 1/2 avocado, chopped

- Bunch of coriander leaves, chopped
- Couple of fresh parsley leaves, chopped
- For your dressing
- 3 tbsp. lime juice
- 1 small garlic clove, finely diced or grated
- 3 tbsp. extra virgin coconut oil (I used 1. tsp. avocado oil and 2 tbsp. Evo)
- 1 tsp. raw honey
- 1/2 tsp. whole grain or Dijon mustard
- 1/2 tsp. sea salt

Directions:

1. Notes: when planning beforehand, dress the salad 10 minutes before serving. The chicken might be substituted with beef chopped, sliced prawns or fish. Vegetarians may use chopped mushrooms or cooked quinoa.
2. Heat the ghee or coconut oil at a tiny skillet pan above medium-high heat. Bring the onion and then sauté on moderate heat for 45 minutes, until golden. Insert the chicken blossom and garlic and simmer for 2-3 minutes on medium-high heat, breaking it all out.
3. Add the garlic, lime zest, lime juice, and salt and soda and cook stirring often, to get a further 3-4 minutes. Place the cooked mince aside.

4. As the chicken is cooking, add a little spoonful of water. Insert the broccoli and cook 2 minutes. Rinse under warm water and then cut into 3-4 pieces each.
5. Insert the pumpkin seeds into the skillet out of the toast and chicken over moderate heat for two minutes, stirring often to avoid burning. Season with a little salt. Set-aside. Raw pumpkin seeds will also be nice to utilize.
6. Put chopped spinach at a salad bowl and then pour over the dressing table. With the hands, massage and toss the carrot with the dressing table. This will dampen the lettuce, a lot similar to what citrus juice will not steak or fish Carpaccio- its "hamburgers" it marginally.
7. Finally, toss throughout the cooked chicken, broccoli, fresh herbs, pumpkin seeds, and avocado pieces.

Nutrition: Calories 166 Fats 13 g Carbohydrates 18 g Proteins 7 g

Buckwheat Noodles with Chicken Kale & Miso Dressing

Preparation time: 15 minutes

Cooking time: 15 minutes

Servings: 2

Ingredients:

For the noodles

- 2 3 handfuls of kale leaves (removed from the stem and fully trimmed)
- 150 g / 5 oz. buckwheat noodles (100 percent buckwheat, no wheat)
- 34 shiitake mushrooms, chopped
- 1 tsp. coconut oil or ghee
- 1 brown onion, finely diced
- 1 moderate free-range chicken, chopped or diced
- 1 red chili, thinly chopped (seeds out based on how hot you want it)
- 2 large garlic cloves, finely-chopped
- 23 tbsp. tamari sauce (fermented soy sauce)

For your miso dressing

- 1 ½ tbsp. fresh organic miso
- 1 tbsp. tamari sauce
- 1 tbsp. peppermint oil
- 1 tbsp. lime or lemon juice
- 1 tsp. sesame oil (optional)

Directions:

1. Bring a medium saucepan of water. Insert the kale and cook 1 minute, until slightly wilted. Remove and put aside but keep the water and put it back to boil. Insert the soba noodles and cook according to the package directions (usually about five minutes). Rinse under warm water and place aside.
2. Meanwhile, pan press the shiitake mushrooms at just a very little ghee or coconut oil (about a tsp.) for 23 minutes, until lightly browned on each side. Sprinkle with sea salt and then place aside.
3. In the exact skillet, warm olive oil ghee over medium-high heating system. Sauté onion and simmer for 2 3 minutes and add the chicken bits. Cook five minutes over medium heat, stirring a few days, you can put in the garlic, tamari sauce and just a tiny dab of water. Cook for a further 2-3 minutes, stirring often until chicken is cooked through.
4. Last, add the carrot and soba noodles and chuck throughout the chicken to heat up.
5. Mix the miso dressing and scatter on the noodles before eating; in this manner, you can retain dozens of enzymes that are beneficial at the miso.

Nutrition: 342 Calories

Asian King Prawn Stir Fry Together with Buckwheat Noodles

Preparation time: 10 minutes

Cooking time: 8 minutes

Servings: 1

Ingredients:

- 150g shelled raw king prawns, deveined
- Two tsp. tamari (it is possible to utilize soy sauce in the event that you aren't quitting gluten)
- Two tsp. extra virgin coconut oil
- 75g soba (buckwheat noodles)
- 1 garlic clove, finely chopped
- 1 bird's-eye chili, finely chopped
- 1 tsp. finely chopped ginger
- 20g red onions, chopped
- 40g celery, trimmed and chopped
- 75g green beans, sliced
- 50g kale, approximately sliced
- 100ml poultry inventory
- 5g lovage or celery leaves

Directions:

1. Heating a skillet on high heat, cook the prawns into 1 tsp. of this tamari and one tsp. of the oil 2--three minutes. Transfer the prawns into your plate. Wipe out the pan with kitchen paper, even because you are going to make use of it.
2. Cook the noodles in boiling water --8 minutes as directed on the package. Drain and put aside.
3. Meanwhile, squeeze the garlic, chili and ginger, red onion, celery, lettuce and beans at the rest of the oil over medium-high temperature for two-three minutes. Bring the stock and bring to the boil, then simmer for a moment or two, before the veggies have been cooked but still crunchy.
4. Insert both the prawns, noodles and lovage/celery leaves into the pan, then return to the boil and then remove from heat and serve.

Nutrition: 340 calories

Dessert Recipes – Phase 1

Creamy Strawberry & Cherry Smoothie

Preparation time: 20 Minutes

Cooking time: 0 Minutes

Servings: 2

Ingredients:

- 100g 3½ oz. strawberries
- 75g 3oz. frozen pitted cherries
- 1 tablespoon plain full-fat yogurt
- 175mls 6fl oz. unsweetened soya milk
- 132 calories per serving

Directions:

1. Place all of the ingredients into a blender and process until smooth. Serve and enjoy.

Nutrition: 254 Cal

Grape, Celery & Parsley Reviver

Preparation time: 10 Minutes

Cooking time: 0 Minutes

Servings: 2

Ingredients:

- 75g 3ozred grapes
- 3 sticks of celery
- 1 avocado, de-stoned and peeled
- 1 tablespoon fresh parsley
- ½ teaspoon Matcha powder
- 334 calories per serving

Directions:

1. Place all of the ingredients into a blender with enough water to cover them and blitz until smooth and creamy. Add crushed ice to make it even more refreshing.

Nutrition: 275 calories

Strawberry & Citrus Blend

Preparation time: 20 Minutes

Cooking time: 0 Minutes

Servings: 2

Ingredients:

- 75g 3ozstrawberries
- 1 apple, cored
- 1 orange, peeled
- ½ avocado, peeled and de-stoned
- ½ teaspoon Matcha powder
- Juice of 1 lime

Directions:

1. Place all of the ingredients into a blender with enough water to cover them and process until smooth.

Nutrition: 272 calories per serving

Chocolate Hazelnut Brownie Pie

Preparation time: 10 minutes

Cooking time: 30 minutes

Servings: 8

Ingredients:

- ¾ cup of granulated Erythritol-based Sweetener
- 4 oz. of coarsely chopped unsweetened Chocolate
- 4 large eggs
- ½ cup of boiling Water
- 1 tsp. Vanilla extract
- 100g (1 cup) Hazelnut meal
- 1 stick (½ cups) unsalted Butter

Directions:

1. Heat the oven to 350° F. Grease a 9-inch ceramic pie pan or glass.
2. Pulse the sweetener and the chopped chocolate in a food processor. Carefully pour in boiling water while the food processor is running on high until the chocolate becomes smooth and melted.
3. Add the vanilla extract, butter, and eggs and process until it is well mixed. Fold in the hazelnut and process to make sure it well combined.
4. Pour batter into greased pan and bake for 25-30 minutes so that the middle becomes somewhat wet but the sides becomes finely set. Take it out of the oven and cool. Refrigerate for 2 hours.
5. Garnish with toasted hazelnuts and whipped cream.

Nutrition: Fat: 28.4g Carbs: 6.8g Protein: 7.3g Calories: 324

Dessert Recipes – Phase 1

Slice-and-Bake Vanilla Wafers

Preparation time: 10 minutes

Cooking time: 15 minutes

Servings: 2

Ingredients:

- 175g (1¾ cups) blanched Almond flour
- ½ cup granulated Erythritol-based Sweetener
- 1 stick (½ cup) unsalted softened Butter
- 2 tbsp. of Coconut flour
- ¼ tsp. of salt
- ½ tsp. of Vanilla extract

Directions:

1. Beat the sweetener and butter using an electric mixer in a large bowl for 2 minutes until it becomes fluffy and light. Then beat in the salt, vanilla extract, coconut flour, and almond until thoroughly mixed.
2. Evenly spread the dough between two sheets of parchment or wax paper and wrap each portion into a size with a diameter of about 1½ inches. Then wrap in paper and refrigerate for 1-2 hours.
3. Heat the oven to 325° F and line a baking sheet using silicone baking mats or parchment paper. Slice the dough into ¼- inch slices using a sharp knife. Put the sliced dough on the baking sheets and make sure to leave a 1-inch space between wafers.
4. Place in the oven for about 5 minutes. Slightly flatten the cookies using a flat-bottomed glass. Bake for another 8-10 minutes.

Nutrition: Protein: 2.2g Fat: 9.3g Carbs: 2.5g Calories: 101

Amaretti

Preparation time: 15 minutes

Cooking time: 22 minutes

Servings: 2

Ingredients:

- ½ cup of granulated Erythritol-based Sweetener
- 165g (2 cups) sliced Almonds
- ¼ cup of powdered of Erythritol-based sweetener
- 4 large egg whites
- Pinch of salt
- ½ tsp. almond extract

Directions:

1. Heat the oven to 300° F and use parchment paper to line 2 baking sheets. Grease the parchment slightly.
2. Process the powdered sweetener, granulated sweetener, and sliced almonds in a food processor until it appears like coarse crumbs.
3. Beat the egg whites plus the salt and almond extracts using an electric mixer in a large bowl until they hold soft peaks. Fold in the almond mixture so that it becomes well combined.
4. Drop spoonful of the dough onto the prepared baking sheet and allow for a space of 1 inch between them. Press a sliced almond into the top of each cookie.
5. Bake in the oven for 22 minutes until the sides becomes brown. They will appear jellylike when they are taken out from the oven but will begin to be firms as it cools down.

Nutrition: Fat: 8.8g Carbs: 4.1g Protein: 5.3g Calories: 117

Peanut Butter Cookies for Two

Preparation time: 5 minutes

Cooking time: 12 minutes

Servings: 1

Ingredients:

- 1½ tbsp. of creamy salted Peanut Butter
- 1 tbsp. of unsalted softened Butter
- 2 tsp. of lightly beaten egg
- 2 tbsp. of granulated Erythritol-based Sweetener
- ¼ tsp. of Vanilla extract
- 2 tbsp. of defatted Peanut flour
- Pinch of salt
- 2 tsp. of sugarless Chocolate Chips
- ⅛ Tsp. of baking powder

Directions:

1. Heat the oven to 325° F and line a baking sheet with a silicone baking mat or parchment paper.
2. Beat in the sweetener, butter, and peanut butter using an electric mixer in a small bowl until it is thoroughly mixed. Then beat in the vanilla extract and the egg.
3. Add the salt, baking powder, and peanut flour and mix until the dough clumps together. Cut the dough into two and shape each of them into a ball.
4. Position the dough ball into the coated baking sheets and flatten into a circular shape about ½ inches thick. Garnish the dough tops with a tsp. of chocolate chips. Gently press them into the dough to stick.
5. Bake for 10-12 minutes until golden brown.

Nutrition: Fat: 13.2g Carbs: 5.7g Protein: 4.9g Calories: 163

Cream Cheese Cookies

Preparation time: 15 minutes

Cooking time: 12 minutes

Servings: 6

Ingredients:

- ¼ cup (½ stick) unsalted softened Butter
- ½ cup (4 oz.) of softened Cream Cheese
- 1 large egg at room temp
- ½ of cup granulated Erythritol-based Sweetener
- 150g (1½ cups) of blanched Almond flour
- 1 tsp. of baking Powder
- ½ tsp. of Vanilla extract
- Powdered Erythritol-based sweetener (for dusting)
- ¼ tsp. of salt

Directions:

1. Heat the oven to 350°F and line with a silicone baking mat or parchment paper.
2. Beat the butter and cream cheese using an electric mixer in a large bowl until it appears smooth. Add the sweetener and keep beating. Beat in the vanilla extract and the egg.
3. Whisk in the salt, baking powder, and almond flour in a medium bowl. Add the flour mixture into the cream cheese and until well incorporated.
4. Drop the dough in spoonful onto the coated baking sheet. Flatten the cookies.
5. Bake for 10-12 minutes. Dust with powdered sweetener when cool.

Nutrition: Fat: 13.7g Carbs: 3.4g Protein: 4.1gCalories: 154

Chewy Double Chocolate Cookies

Preparation time: 15 minutes

Cooking time: 12 minutes

Servings: 10

Ingredients:

- 3 tbsp. of Cocoa powder
- 2 tbsp. of (88g) plus ¾ cup blanched Almond flour
- ½ tsp. of baking soda
- 1 tbsp. of grass-fed Gelatin
- ½ tsp. of salt
- ½ stick (¼ cup) unsalted softened Butter
- ½ cup of granulated Erythritol-based sweetener
- 1 large egg at room temp
- ¼ cup of unsalted Creamy Almond Butter
- ½ tsp. of Vanilla extract
- ⅓ cup sugarless Chocolate Chips

Directions:

1. Heat the oven to 350° F and line 2 baking sheets with silicone baking mats or parchment paper.
2. Whisk the gelatin, salt, baking soda, cocoa powder, and almond flour together in a medium bowl.
3. Beat the sweetener, almond butter, and butter with an electric mixer in a large bowl until it is thoroughly mixed. Beat the vanilla extract and the egg. The beat in the almond mixture so that the dough sticks together. Add the chocolate chips and stir.
4. Roll the dough into medium-sized cookies and space them an inch apart. Flatten to about ½ inch thick
5. Bake for about 12 minutes.

Nutrition: Fat: 15.1g Carbs: 6.9g Protein: 5.5g Calories: 180

Mocha Cream Pie

Preparation time: 15 minutes

Cooking time: 5 minutes

Servings: 10

Ingredients:

- 1 cup strongly brewed Coffee at room temp
- 1 Easy Chocolate Pie Crust
- 1 cup heavy Whipping Cream
- 1½ tsp. of grass-fed Gelatin
- 1 tsp. of Vanilla extract
- ¼ cup Cocoa powder
- ½ cup powdered Erythritol-based Sweetener

Directions:

1. Grease a 9-inch glass pie pan or ceramic. Press the crust mixture evenly and firmly to the sides of the greased pan or its bottom. Refrigerate until the filling is prepared.
2. Pour the coffee in a small saucepan and add gelatin. Whisk thoroughly and then place over medium heat. Allow simmering, whisking from time to time to make sure the gelatin dissolves. Allow to cool for 20 minutes.
3. Add the vanilla extract, cocoa powder, sweetener, and the cream into a large bowl. Use an electric mixer to beat to that it holds stiff peaks.
4. Add gelatin mixture that has been cooled and then beat until it is well incorporated. Pour over the cooled crust and place in the refrigerator for 3 hours until it becomes firm.

Nutrition: Fat: 20.2g Carbs: 6.2g Protein: 4.7g Calories: 218

Coconut Custard Pie

Preparation time: 10 minutes

Cooking time: 50 minutes

Servings: 8

Ingredients:

- 1 cup of heavy Whipping Cream
- ¾ cup of powdered Erythritol-based Sweetener
- ½ cup of full-fat Coconut Milk
- 4 large eggs
- ½ stick (¼ cup) of cooled, unsalted, melted butter
- 1¼ cups of unsweetened shredded coconut
- 3 tbsp. of Coconut flour
- ½ tsp. of baking powder
- ½ tsp. of Vanilla extract
- ¼ tsp. of salt

Directions:

1. Heat the oven to 350° F and grease a 9-inch ceramic pie pan or glass.
2. Place the melted butter, eggs, coconut milk, sweetener, and cream in a blender. Blend well.
3. Add the vanilla extract, baking powder, salt, coconut flour, and a cup of shredded coconut. Continue blending.
4. Empty the mixture into the pie pan and sprinkle with the rest of the shredded coconut. Bake for 40-50 minutes and stop when the center is until jiggly but the sides are set.
5. Take out of the oven and allow it to cool for 30 minutes. Place in the refrigerator and allow staying for 2 hours before cutting it.

Nutrition: Fat: 29.5g Carbs: 6.7g Protein: 5.3g Calories: 317

Dairy-Free Fruit Tarts

Preparation time: 15 minutes

Cooking time: 15 minutes

Servings: 2

Ingredients:

- 1 cup Coconut Whipped Cream
- ½ Easy Shortbread Crust (dairy-free option)
- Fresh mint Sprigs
- ½ cup mixed fresh Berries

Directions:

1. Grease two 4" pans with detachable bottoms. Pour the shortbread mixture into pans and firmly press into the edges and bottom of each pan. Refrigerate for 15 minutes.
2. Loosen the crust carefully to remove from the pan.
3. Distribute the whipped cream between the tarts and evenly spread to the sides. Refrigerate for 1-2 hours to make it firm.
4. Use the berries and sprig of mint to garnish each of the tarts

Nutrition: Fat: 28.9g Carbs: 8.3g Protein: 5.8g Calories: 306

Dessert Recipes – Phase 1

Other Recipes – Phase1

Apple & Celery Juice

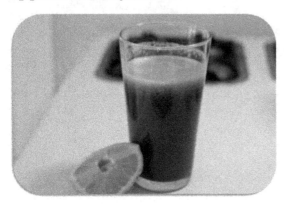

Preparation time: 10 minutes

Cooking time: 0 minutes

Servings: 2

Ingredients:

- 4 large green apples, cored and sliced
- 4 celery stalks
- 1 lemon, peeled

Directions:

1. Add all ingredients into a juicer and extract the juice according to the manufacturer's method.
2. Pour into 2 glasses and serve immediately.

Nutrition: Calories 240 Total Fat 0.9 g Saturated Fat 0 g Cholesterol 0 mg Protein 1.5 g

Broccoli, Apple, & Orange Juice

Preparation time: 10 minutes

Cooking time: 0 minutes

Servings: 2

Ingredients:

- 2 broccoli stalks, chopped
- 2 large green apples, cored and sliced
- 3 large oranges, peeled and sectioned
- 4 tablespoons fresh parsley

Directions:

1. Add all ingredients into a juicer and extract the juice according to the manufacturer's method.
2. Pour into 2 glasses and serve immediately.

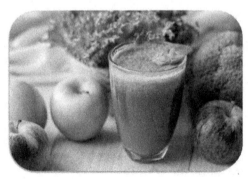

Nutrition: Calories 254 Total Fat 0.8 g Saturated Fat 0.1 g Protein 3.8 g

Green Fruit Juice

Preparation time: 10 minutes

Cooking time: 0 minutes

Servings: 2

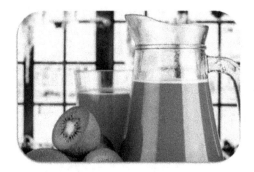

Ingredients:

- 3 large kiwis, peeled and chopped
- 3 large green apples, cored and sliced
- 2 cups seedless green grapes
- 2 teaspoons fresh lime juice

Directions:

1. Add all ingredients into a juicer and extract the juice according to the manufacturer's method.
2. Pour into 2 glasses and serve immediately.

Nutrition: Calories 304 Total Fat 2.2 g Saturated Fat 0 g Protein 6.2 g

Kale & Fruit Juice

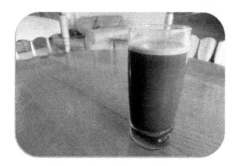

Preparation time: 10 minutes

Cooking time: 0 minutes

Servings: 2

Ingredients:

- 2 large green apples, cored and sliced
- 2 large pears, cored and sliced
- 3 cups fresh kale leaves
- 3 celery stalks
- 1 lemon, peeled

Directions:

1. Add all ingredients into a juicer and extract the juice according to the manufacturer's method.
2. Pour into 2 glasses and serve immediately.

Nutrition: Calories 293 Total Fat 0.8 g Saturated Fat 0 g Cholesterol 0 mg Protein 4.6 g

Kale, Carrot, & Grapefruit Juice

Preparation time: 10 minutes

Cooking time: 0 minutes

Servings: 2

Ingredients:

- 3 cups fresh kale
- 2 large Granny Smith apples, cored and sliced
- 2 medium carrots, peeled and chopped
- 2 medium grapefruit, peeled and sectioned
- 1 teaspoon fresh lemon juice

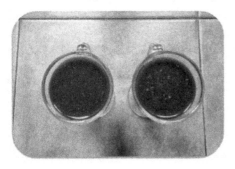

Directions:

1. Add all ingredients into a juicer and extract the juice according to the manufacturer's method.
2. Pour into 2 glasses and serve immediately.

Nutrition: Calories 232 Total Fat 0.6 g Saturated Fat 0 g Cholesterol 0 mg Protein 4.9 g

Buckwheat Granola

Preparation time: 15 minutes

Cooking time: 30 minutes

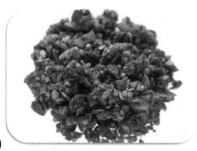

Servings: 10

Ingredients:

- 2 cups raw buckwheat groats
- ¾ cup pumpkin seeds
- ¾ cup almonds, chopped
- 1 cup unsweetened coconut flakes
- 1 teaspoon ground cinnamon
- 1 teaspoon ground ginger
- 1 ripe banana, peeled
- 2 tablespoons maple syrup
- 2 tablespoons olive oil

Directions:

1. Preheat your oven to 350ºF.
2. In a bowl, place the buckwheat groats, coconut flakes, pumpkin seeds, almonds, and spices, and mix well.
3. In another bowl, add the banana and with a fork, mash well.

4. Add to the buckwheat mixture maple syrup and oil, and mix until well combined.
5. Transfer the mixture onto the prepared baking sheet and spread in an even layer.
6. Bake for about 25–30 minutes, stirring once halfway through.
7. Remove the baking sheet from oven and set aside to cool.

Nutrition: Calories 252 Total Fat 14.3 g Saturated Fat 3.7 g Cholesterol 0 mg Protein 7.6 g

Apple Pancakes

Preparation time: 15 minutes

Cooking time: 24 minutes

Servings: 6

Ingredients:

- ½ cup buckwheat flour
- 2 tablespoons coconut sugar
- 1 teaspoon baking powder
- ½ teaspoon ground cinnamon
- 1/3 cup unsweetened almond milk
- 1 egg, beaten lightly
- 2 granny smith apples, peeled, cored, and grated

Directions:

1. In a bowl, place the flour, coconut sugar, and cinnamon, and mix well.
2. In another bowl, place the almond milk and egg and beat until well combined.
3. Now, place the flour mixture and mix until well combined.
4. Fold in the grated apples.
5. Heat a lightly greased non-stick wok over medium-high heat.
6. Add desired amount of mixture and with a spoon, spread into an even layer.

7. Cook for 1-2 minutes on each side.
8. Repeat with the remaining mixture.
9. Serve warm with the drizzling of honey.

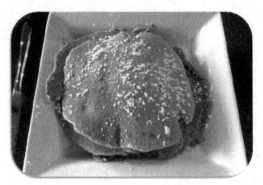

Nutrition: Calories 93 Total Fat 2.1 g Saturated Fat 1 g Cholesterol 27 mg Sugar 12.1 g Protein 2.5 g

Matcha Pancakes

Preparation time: 15 minutes

Cooking time: 24 minutes

Servings: 6

Ingredients:

- 2 tablespoons flax meal
- 5 tablespoons warm water
- 1 cup spelt flour
- 1 cup buckwheat flour
- 1 tablespoon Matcha powder
- 1 tablespoon baking powder
- Pinch of salt
- ¾ cup unsweetened almond milk
- 1 tablespoon olive oil
- 1 teaspoon vanilla extract
- 1/3 cup raw honey

Directions:

1. In a bowl, add the flax meal and warm water and mix well. Set aside for about 5 minutes.

2. In another bowl, place the flours, Matcha powder, baking powder, and salt, and mix well.
3. In the bowl of flax meal mixture, place the almond milk, oil, and vanilla extract, and beat until well combined.
4. Now, place the flour mixture and mix until a smooth textured mixture is formed.
5. Heat a lightly greased non-stick wok over medium-high heat.
6. Add desired amount of mixture and with a spoon, spread into an even layer.
7. Cook for about 2–3 minutes.
8. Carefully, flip the side and cook for about 1 minute.
9. Repeat with the remaining mixture.
10. Serve warm with the drizzling of honey.

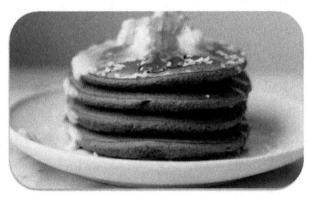

Nutrition: Calories 232 Total Fat 4.6 g Saturated Fat 0.6 g Cholesterol 0 mg Protein 6 g

Smoked Salmon & Kale Scramble

Preparation time: 10 minutes

Cooking time: 9 minutes

Servings: 3

Ingredients:

- 2 cups fresh kale, tough ribs removed and chopped finely
- 1 tablespoon coconut oil
- Ground black pepper, to taste
- ½ cup smoked salmon, crumbled
- 4 eggs, beaten

Directions:

1. In a wok, melt the coconut oil over high heat and cook the kale with black pepper for about 3-4 minutes.
2. Stir in the smoked salmon and reduce the heat to medium.
3. Add the eggs and cook for about 3-4 minutes, stirring frequently.
4. Serve immediately.

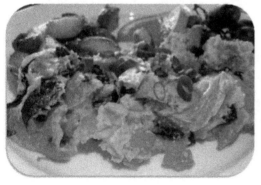

Nutrition: Calories 257 Total Fat 17 g Saturated Fat 8.9 g Cholesterol 335 mg Protein 19.3 g

Kale & Mushroom Frittata

Preparation time: 15 minutes

Cooking time: 30 minutes

Servings: 5

Ingredients:

- 8 eggs
- ½ cup unsweetened almond milk
- Salt and ground black pepper, to taste
- 1 tablespoon olive oil
- 1 onion, chopped
- 1 garlic clove, minced
- 1 cup fresh mushrooms, chopped
- 1½ cups fresh kale, tough ribs removed and chopped

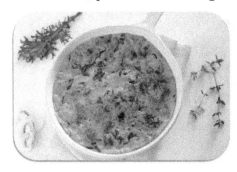

Directions:

1. Preheat oven to 350ºF.
2. In a large bowl, place the eggs, coconut milk, salt, and black pepper, and beat well. Set aside.

3. In a large ovenproof wok, heat the oil over medium heat and sauté the onion and garlic for about 3-4 minutes.
4. Add the squash, kale, bell pepper, salt, and black pepper, and cook for about 8-10 minutes.
5. Stir in the mushrooms and cook for about 3-4 minutes.
6. Add the kale and cook for about 5 minutes.
7. Place the egg mixture on top evenly and cook for about 4 minutes, without stirring.
8. Transfer the wok in the oven and bake for about 12-15 minutes or until desired doneness.
9. Remove from the oven and place the frittata side for about 3-5 minutes before serving.
10. Cut into desired sized wedges and serve.

Nutrition: Calories 151 Total Fat 10.2 g Saturated Fat 2.6 g Cholesterol 262 mg Protein 10.3 g

Kale, Apple, & Cranberry Salad

Preparation time: 15 minutes

Cooking time: 15minutes

Servings: 4

Ingredients:

- 6 cups fresh baby kale
- 3 large apples, cored and sliced
- ¼ cup unsweetened dried cranberries
- ¼ cup almonds, sliced
- 2 tablespoons extra-virgin olive oil
- 1 tablespoon raw honey
- Salt and ground black pepper, to taste

Directions:

1. In a salad bowl, place all the ingredients and toss to coat well.
2. Serve immediately.

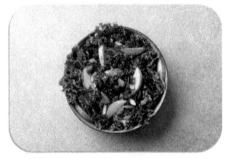

Nutrition: Calories 253 Total Fat 10.3 g Saturated Fat 1.2 g Cholesterol 0 mg Protein 4.7 g

Arugula, Strawberry, & Orange Salad

Preparation time: 15 minutes

Cooking time: 15 minutes

Servings: 4

Ingredients:

Salad:

- 6 cups fresh baby arugula
- 1½ cups fresh strawberries, hulled and sliced
- 2 oranges, peeled and segmented

Dressing:

- 2 tablespoons fresh lemon juice
- 1 tablespoon raw honey
- 2 teaspoons extra-virgin olive oil
- 1 teaspoon Dijon mustard
- Salt and ground black pepper, to taste

Directions:

1. For salad: in a salad bowl, place all ingredients and mix.
2. For dressing: place all ingredients in another bowl and beat until well combined.
3. Place dressing on top of salad and toss to coat well.
4. Serve immediately.

Nutrition: Calories 107 Total Fat 2.9 g Saturated Fat 0.4 g Cholesterol 0 mg Protein 2.1 g

Beef & Kale Salad

Preparation time: 15 minutes

Cooking time: 8 minutes

Servings: 2

Ingredients:

Steak

- 2 teaspoons olive oil
- 2 (4-ounce) strip steaks
- Salt and ground black pepper, to taste

Salad

- ¼ cup carrot, peeled and shredded
- ¼ cup cucumber, peeled, seeded, and sliced
- ¼ cup radish, sliced
- ¼ cup cherry tomatoes, halved
- 3 cups fresh kale, tough ribs removed and chopped

Dressing

- 1 tablespoon extra-virgin olive oil
- 1 tablespoon fresh lemon juice
- Salt and ground black pepper, to taste

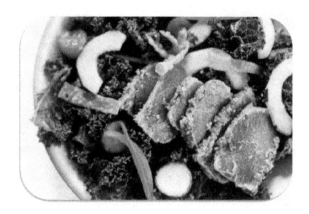

Directions:

1. For steak: in a large heavy-bottomed wok, heat the oil over high heat and cook the steaks with salt and black pepper for about 3–4 minutes per side.
2. Transfer the steaks onto a cutting board for about 5 minutes before slicing.
3. For salad: place all ingredients in a salad bowl and mix.
4. For dressing: place all ingredients in another bowl and beat until well combined.
5. Cut the steaks into desired sized slices against the grain.
6. Place the salad onto each serving plate.
7. Top each plate with steak slices.
8. Drizzle with dressing and serve.

Nutrition: Calories 262 Total Fat 12 g Saturated Fat 1.6 g Protein 25.2 g

Breakfast Recipes – Phase 2

Green Omelette

Preparation time: 10 min

Cooking time: 5 min

Servings: 1

Ingredients:

- 2 large eggs, at room temperature
- 1 shallot, peeled and chopped
- Handful arugula
- 3 sprigs of parsley, chopped
- 1 tsp. extra virgin olive oil
- Salt and black pepper

Directions:

1. Beat the eggs in a small bowl and set aside, sauté the shallot for 5 minutes with a bit of the oil, on low-medium heat. Pour the eggs in the pans, stirring the mixture for just a second.
2. The eggs on a medium heat, and tip the pan just enough to let the loose egg run underneath after about one minute on the burner. Add the greens, herbs, and the seasonings to the top side as it is still soft. TIP: You do not even have to flip it, as you can just cook the egg slowly egg as is well (being careful as to not burn).
3. TIP: Another option is to put it into an oven to broil for 3-5 minutes (checking to make sure it is only until it is golden but burned).

Nutrition: 234 calories

Berry Oat Breakfast Cobbler

Preparation time: 40 min

Cooking time: 5 min

Servings: 2

Ingredients:

- 2 cups of oats/flakes that are ready without cooking
- 1 cup of blackcurrants without the stems
- 1 teaspoon of honey (or ¼ teaspoon of raw sugar)
- ½ cup of water (add more or less by testing the pan)
- 1 cup of plain yogurt (or soy or coconut)

Directions:

1. Boil the berries, honey and water and then turn it down on low. Put in a glass container in a refrigerator until it is cool and set (about 30 minutes or more)
2. When ready to eat, scoop the berries on top of the oats and yogurt. Serve immediately.

Nutrition: 241 calories

Pancakes with Apples and Blackcurrants

Preparation time: 30 min

Cooking time: 10 min

Servings: 4

Ingredients:

- 2 apples, cut into small chunks
- 2 cups of quick cooking oats
- 1 cup flour of your choice
- 1 tsp. baking powder
- 2 tbsp. raw sugar, coconut sugar, or 2 tbsp. honey that is warm and easy to distribute
- 2 egg whites
- 1 ¼ cups of milk (or soy/rice/coconut)
- 2 tsp. extra virgin olive oil
- A dash of salt

For the berry topping:

- 1 cup blackcurrants, washed and stalks removed
- 3 tbsp. water (may use less)
- 2 tbsp. sugar (see above for types)

Directions:

1. Place the ingredients for the topping in a small pot simmer, stirring frequently for about 10 minutes until it cooks down and the juices are released.

2. Take the dry ingredients and mix in a bowl. After, add the apples and the milk a bit at a time (you may not use it all), until it is a batter. Stiffly whisk the egg whites and then gently mix them into the pancake batter. Set aside in the refrigerator.
3. Pour a one quarter of the oil onto a flat pan or flat griddle, and when hot, pour some of the batter into it in a pancake shape. When the pancakes start to have golden brown edges and form air bubbles, they may be ready to be gently flipped.
4. Test to be sure the bottom can life away from the pan before actually flipping. Repeat for the next three pancakes. Top each pancake with the berries.

Nutrition: 337 calories

Granola- The Sirt Way

Preparation time: 30 min

Cooking time: 0 min

Servings: 1

Ingredients:

- 1 cup buckwheat puffs
- 1 cup buckwheat flakes (ready to eat type, but not whole buckwheat that needs to be cooked) ½ cup coconut flakes
- ½ cup Medjool dates, without pits, chopped into smaller, bite-sized pieces
- 1 cup of cacao nibs or very dark chocolate chips
- 1/2 cup walnuts, chopped
- 1 cup strawberries chopped and without stem 1 cup plain Greek, or coconut or soy yogurt.

Directions:

1. Mix, without yogurt and strawberry toppings
2. You can store for up to a week, store in an airtight container. Add toppings (even different berries or different yogurt.
3. You can even use the berry toppings as you will learn how to make from other recipes.

Nutrition: 235 Cal

Summer Berry Smoothie

Preparation time: 30 min

Cooking time: 0 min

Servings: 1

Ingredients

- 50g (2oz) blueberries
- 50g (2oz) strawberries
- 25g (1oz) blackcurrants
- 25g (1oz) red grapes
- 1 carrot, peeled
- 1 orange, peeled
- Juice of 1 lime

Directions:

1. Place all of the ingredients into a blender and cover them with water. Blitz until smooth. You can also add some crushed ice and a mint leaf to garnish.

Nutrition: 300 Cal

Mango, Celery & Ginger Smoothie

Preparation time: 30 min

Cooking time: 0 min

Servings: 1

Ingredients:

- 1 stalk of celery
- 50g (2oz) kale
- 1 apple, cored
- 50g (2oz) mango, peeled, de-stoned and chopped
- 2.5cm (1 inch) chunk of fresh ginger root, peeled and chopped

Directions:

1. Put all the ingredients into a blender with some water and blitz until smooth. Add ice to make your smoothie really refreshing.

Nutrition: 275 Cal

Orange, Carrot & Kale Smoothie

Preparation time: 30 min

Cooking time: 0 min

Servings: 1

Ingredients:

- 1 carrot, peeled
- 1 orange, peeled
- 1 stick of celery
- 1 apple, cored
- 50g (2oz) kale
- ½ teaspoon Matcha powder

Directions:

1. Place all of the ingredients into a blender and add in enough water to cover them. Process until smooth, serve and enjoy.

Nutrition: 279 Cal

Creamy Strawberry & Cherry Smoothie

Preparation time: 30 min

Cooking time: 0 min

Servings: 1

Ingredients:

- 100g (3½ oz.) strawberries
- 75g (3oz) frozen pitted cherries
- 1 tablespoon plain full-fat yogurt
- 175mls (6fl oz.) unsweetened soya milk

Directions:

1. Place all of the ingredients into a blender and process until smooth. Serve and enjoy.

Nutrition: 280 Cal

Grape, Celery & Parsley Reviver

Preparation time: 30 min

Cooking time: 0 min

Servings: 1

Ingredients:

- 75g (3oz) red grapes
- 3 sticks of celery
- 1 avocado, de-stoned and peeled
- 1 tablespoon fresh parsley
- ½ teaspoon Matcha powder

Directions:

1. Place all of the ingredients into a blender with enough water to cover them and blitz until smooth and creamy. Add crushed ice to make it even more refreshing.

Nutrition: 230Cal

Strawberry & Citrus Blend

Preparation time: 30 min

Cooking time: 0 min

Servings: 1

Ingredients:

- 75g (3oz) strawberries
- 1 apple, cored
- 1 orange, peeled
- ½ avocado, peeled and de-stoned
- ½ teaspoon Matcha powder
- Juice of 1 lime

Directions:

1. Place all of the ingredients into a blender with enough water to cover them and process until smooth.

Nutrition: 250 Cal

Grapefruit & Celery Blast

Preparation time: 30 min

Cooking time: 0 min

Servings: 1

Ingredients:

- 1 grapefruit, peeled
- 2 stalks of celery
- 50g (2oz) kale
- ½ teaspoon Matcha powder

Directions:

1. Place all the ingredients into a blender with enough water to cover them and blitz until smooth.

Nutrition: 286 Cal

Orange & Celery Crush

Preparation time: 30 min

Cooking time: 0 min

Servings: 1

Ingredients

- 1 carrot, peeled
- 3 stalks of celery
- 1 orange, peeled
- ½ teaspoon Matcha powder
- Juice of 1 lime

Directions:

1. Place all of the ingredients into a blender with enough water to cover them and blitz until smooth.

Nutrition: 274 Cal

Tropical Chocolate Delight

Preparation time: 30 min

Cooking time: 0 min

Servings: 1

Ingredients:

- 1 mango, peeled & de-stoned
- 75g (3oz) fresh pineapple, chopped
- 50g (2oz) kale
- 25g (1oz) rocket
- 1 tablespoon 100% cocoa powder or cacao nibs
- 150mls (5fl oz.) coconut milk

Directions:

1. Place all of the ingredients into a blender and blitz until smooth. You can add a little water if it seems too thick.

Nutrition: 288 Cal

Walnut & Spiced Apple Tonic

Preparation time: 30 min

Cooking time: 0 min

Servings: 1

Ingredients:

- 6 walnuts halves
- 1 apple, cored
- 1 banana
- ½ teaspoon Matcha powder
- ½ teaspoon cinnamon
- Pinch of ground nutmeg

Directions:

1. Place all of the ingredients into a blender and add sufficient water to cover them, blitz until smooth and creamy.

Nutrition: 258 Cal

Pineapple & Cucumber Smoothie

Preparation time: 30 min

Cooking time: 0 min

Servings: 1

Ingredients:

- 50g (2oz) cucumber
- 1 stalk of celery
- 2 slices of fresh pineapple
- 2 sprigs of parsley
- ½ teaspoon Matcha powder
- Squeeze of lemon juice

Directions:

1. Place all of the ingredients into blender with enough water to cover them and blitz until smooth.

Nutrition: 260 Cal

Breakfast Recipes – Phase 2

Main Meals Recipes – Phase 2

Honey Chili Squash

Preparation time: 5 Minutes

Cooking time: 50 Minutes

Servings: 2

Ingredients:

- 2 red onions, roughly chopped 2.5cm
- 1-inch chunk of ginger root, finely chopped
- 2 cloves of garlic
- 2 bird's-eye chilies, finely chopped
- 1 butternut squash, peeled and chopped
- 100 ml 3½ fl. oz. vegetable stock broth
- 1 tablespoon olive oil
- Juice of 1 orange
- Juice of 1 lime
- 2 teaspoons honey

Directions:

1. Warm the oil into a pan and add in the red onions, squash chunks, chilies, garlic, ginger and honey. Cook for 3 minutes. Squeeze in the lime and orange juice. Pour in the stock broth), orange and lime juice and cook for 15 minutes until tender.

Nutrition: 118 calories per serving

Chicken & Bean Casserole

Preparation time: 5 Minutes

Cooking time: 40 Minutes

Servings: 2

Ingredients:

- 400g 14oz chopped tomatoes
- 400g 14 oz. tinned cannellini beans or haricot beans
- 8 chicken thighs, skin removed
- 2 carrots, peeled and finely chopped
- 2 red onions, chopped
- 4 sticks of celery
- 4 large mushrooms
- 2 red peppers bell peppers, deseeded and chopped
- 1 clove of garlic
- 2 tablespoons soy sauce
- 1 tablespoon olive oil
- 1.75 liters 3 pints chicken stock broth

Directions:

1. Heat the olive oil in a saucepan, add the garlic and onions and cook for 5 minutes. Add in the chicken and cook for 5 minutes then add the carrots, cannellini beans, celery, red peppers bell peppers and mushrooms. Pour in the stock broth soy sauce and tomatoes. Bring it to the boil, reduce the heat and simmer for 45 minutes. Serve with rice or new potatoes.

Nutrition: 509 calories per serving

Roast Balsamic Vegetables

Preparation time: 5 Minutes

Cooking time: 45 Minutes

Servings: 2

Ingredients:

- 4 tomatoes, chopped
- 2 red onions, chopped
- 3 sweet potatoes, peeled and chopped
- 100g 3½ oz. red chicory or if unavailable, use yellow
- 100g 3½ oz. kale, finely chopped
- 300g 11oz potatoes, peeled and chopped
- 5 stalks of celery, chopped
- 1 bird's-eye chili, de-seeded and finely chopped
- 2 tablespoons fresh parsley, chopped
- 2 tablespoons fresh coriander cilantro chopped
- 3 tablespoons olive oil
- 2 tablespoons balsamic vinegar 1 teaspoon mustard
- Sea salt
- Freshly ground black pepper

Directions:

1. Place the olive oil, balsamic, mustard, parsley and coriander cilantro into a bowl and mix well. Toss all the remaining ingredients into the dressing and season with salt and pepper. Transfer the vegetables to an ovenproof dish and cook in the oven at 200C/400F for 45 minutes.

Nutrition: 310 calories per serving

Mussels in Red Wine Sauce

Preparation time: 5 Minutes

Cooking time: 50 Minutes

Servings: 2

Ingredients:

- 800g 2lb mussels
- 2 x 400g 14 oz. tins of chopped tomatoes
- 25g 1oz butter
- 1 tablespoon fresh chives, chopped
- 1 tablespoon fresh parsley, chopped
- 1 bird's-eye chili, finely chopped
- 4 cloves of garlic, crushed
- 400 ml 14fl. oz. red wine
- Juice of 1 lemon

Directions:

1. Wash the mussels, remove their beards and set them aside. Heat the butter in a large saucepan and add in the red wine. Reduce the heat and add the parsley, chives, chili and garlic whilst stirring. Add in the tomatoes, lemon juice and mussels. Cover the saucepan and cook for 2-3 minutes. Remove the saucepan from the heat and take out any mussels which haven't opened and discard them. Serve and eat immediately.

Nutrition: 364 calories per serving

Main Meals Recipes – Phase 2 (Part 2)

Courgette Risotto

Preparation time: 10 minutes

Cooking time: 5 minutes

Servings: 8

Ingredients:

- 2 tablespoons olive oil
- 4 cloves garlic, finely chopped
- j1.5 pounds Arborio rice
- 6 tomatoes, chopped
- 2 teaspoons chopped rosemary
- 6 courgettes, finely diced
- 1 ¼ cups peas, fresh or frozen
- 12 cups hot vegetable stock
- 1 cup chopped
- Salt to taste
- Freshly ground pepper

Directions:

1. Place a large heavy bottomed pan over medium heat. Add oil. When the oil is heated, add onion and sauté until translucent.
2. Stir in the tomatoes and cook until soft.
3. Next stir in the rice and rosemary, mix well.
4. Add half the stock and cook until dry. Stir frequently.
5. Add remaining stock and cook for 3-4 minutes.
6. Add courgette and peas and cook until rice is tender. Add salt and pepper to taste.
7. Stir in the basil. Let it sit for 5 minutes.

Nutrition: Calories 406 Fats 5 g Carbohydrates 82 g Proteins 14 g

Chilli Con Carne

Preparation time: 10 minutes

Cooking time: 20 minutes

Servings: 8

Ingredients:

- 1 tsp. hot chilli powder
- 1 tsp. paprika
- 1 large onion
- 2 tbsp. tomato purée
- 1 red pepper
- 1 tsp. ground cumin
- 1 tbsp. oil
- 1 beef stock cube
- 2 garlic cloves
- 1 tsp. sugar (you can also add a little piece of dark chocolate)
- 410g can red kidney beans
- 400g can chopped tomatoes
- 500g minced beef
- ½ tsp. dried marjoram
- Plain boiled long grain rice, to serve
- Soured cream, to serve

Directions:

1. Have your vegetables prepared. Chop into tiny dice 1 big onion, around 5 mm long. The best way to achieve so is to split the onion in half, peel it and then slice it lengthwise into a shape of thick matchsticks every second, not

Main Meals Recipes – Phase 2 (Part 2)

chopping them all to the root end because they are all kept together, round into dice over the match sticks.
2. Slice a red pepper in the half lengthwise, cut base, wash off the seeds, and then chop it. Then peel and cut 2 cloves of garlic.
3. Start off preparation. Place your pan over medium heat onto the hob. Apply 1 tbsp. of oil and keep on for 1 or 2 minutes before heated (if you use an electric hob a little longer).
4. Put the onion and cook for around 5 minutes, stirring relatively regularly, or until your onion is thick, squidgy and somewhat translucent.
5. Tip the 1 tsp. of hot chili powder or you can also add 1 tbsp. of soft chili powder, garlic, red pepper, and 1 tsp. of paprika then 1 tsp. of cumin ground.
6. Offer it a quick swirl, then leave for more 5 minutes to cook, stirring periodically.
7. Brown 500 g lean beef in a minced form, switch the flame up a little, add your meat to the saucepan and split it with the spatula or knife. When you insert the mince, the blend will sizzle a little bit.
8. Keep mixing and prodding for 5 minutes at least, before all mince thing is in place, thin lumps and no pink parts are left. Keep your heat hot enough to fry the meat and turn brown, rather to just stewing.
9. Create a sauce. Crumble 1 cube of beef reserve into 300ml of hot broth. Pour it in the mixture being minced into the pan.
10. Add chopped tomatoes to a 400 g bowl. Top with 1/2 tsp. of dried marjoram, 1 tsp. of sugar and then add a good pepper and salt shake. Sprinkle with some 2 tbsp. of tomato purée and then stir well the sauce.

11. Simmer softly around it. Bring the whole to the boil, stir well and put a cover on the saucepan. Shift the heat down until it spills softly, then quit for almost 20 minutes.
12. Occasionally check on the skillet to mix it, to be sure that the sauce does not stick on the bottom of the pan or dried out. If so, apply a couple tablespoons of water, and ensure that the heat is very small enough. The saucy, minced mixture should look moist, thick and juicy after gently simmering.
13. Drain and then rinse in a sieve a 410 g can of your kidney beans, then mix them into chili pot. Boil again, and bubble gently for more 10 minutes without the lid, you can add a little water more if it looks dry.
14. Taste a little of the season and chilli. Possibly, it would require far much seasoning than you thought.
15. Now remove the cover, turn off the flame and allow the chilli to remain until serving for about10 minutes. This is very important because it requires blending of the flavors.
16. Serve with simple boiled large grain rice and some soured cream.

Nutrition: Calories 403 Fats 4 g Carbohydrates 90 g Proteins 10 g

Brown Basmati Rice Pilaf

Preparation time: 10 minutes

Cooking time: 3 minutes

Servings: 2

Ingredients:

- ½ tablespoon vegan butter
- ½ cup mushrooms, chopped
- ½ cup brown basmati rice
- 2-3 tablespoons water
- 1/8 teaspoon dried thyme
- Ground pepper to taste
- ½ tablespoon olive oil
- ¼ cup green onion, chopped
- 1 cup vegetable broth
- ¼ teaspoon salt
- ¼ cup chopped, toasted pecans

Directions:

1. Place a saucepan over medium-low heat. Add butter and oil.
2. When it melts, add mushrooms and cook until slightly tender.
3. Stir in the green onion and brown rice. Cook for 3 minutes. Stir constantly.
4. Stir in the broth, water, salt and thyme.
5. When it begins to boil, lower heat and cover with a lid. Simmer until rice is cooked. Add more water or broth if required.
6. Stir in the pecans and pepper. Serve

Nutrition: Calories 189 Fats 11 g Carbohydrates 19 g Proteins 4 g

Thai Red Curry

Preparation time: 15 minutes

Cooking time: 1 hour

Servings: 4

Ingredients:

- 1 ½ cups packed thinly sliced kale
- Pinch of salt, more to taste
- 2 tablespoons Thai red curry paste
- 1 tablespoon soy sauce
- 1 ¼ cups long-grain brown jasmine rice
- 1 small white onion, chopped
- 1 tablespoon grated ginger
- 1 red bell pepper
- 1 tablespoon coconut oil or olive oil
- ½ cup water
- 1 ½ teaspoons of coconut sugar or turbinado sugar
- 2 cloves garlic
- 2 of teaspoons lime juice
- 3 carrots, peeled and sliced
- 1 bell pepper
- 1 can (14 ounces) regular coconut milk

Directions:

1. Take a big pot of water and put it to boil to prepare the rice. Insert the rinsed rice and start to boil for 30 minutes to avoid excess, decreasing heat when required. Remove from heat, drain rice, and put the rice back into the pot. Cover and let the rice rest until you are ready to serve for 10 minutes or longer. Season the rice to taste with salt just before serving, and fluff it with a fork.

2. To render the curry, fire up a broad skillet over medium fire with the deep sides, once warm, add your oil. Then add the onion and a sprinkle of salt and cook, stirring frequently for about 5 minutes until your onion has softened and turns translucent. Add the garlic and ginger, and cook for about 25-30 seconds while continuously stirring until fragrant.
3. Add the carrots and your bell peppers, cook, stirring regularly, until these bell peppers are fork-tender, 3 to 5 minutes more. Then add your curry paste, and cook for about 2 minutes, stirring frequently.
4. Add the water, kale, coconut milk, and sugar and whisk to mix. Bring in the mixture over medium flame to a simmer. Reduce flame as needed to keep a mild simmer and cook until the carrots, peppers, and kale have softened to your liking, stirring occasionally for about 5-10 minutes.
5. Remove your pot from flame and season with rice vinegar and tamari. Add salt (for optimum flavor), to taste. If your curry requires a little of more energy, add 1/2 teaspoon more tamari, or add 1/2 teaspoon more of your rice vinegar for more acidity. Divide both curry and rice into bowls and garnish them, if you like, with sliced cilantro and a sprinkle of your red pepper flakes. Serve on the side with sriracha or chili garlic sauce, if you like spicy curries.
6. If you want to add Tofu, first bake it and add it with coconut milk in step 4. If you apply raw tofu, it will take up so much of the fat, so baking it would enhance the flavor considerably, anyway.

Nutrition: Calories 133 Fats 15 g Carbohydrates 17 g Proteins 6 g

Artichoke & Eggplant Rice

Preparation time: 5 minutes

Cooking time: 10 minutes

Servings: 3

Ingredients:

- 2 tablespoons olive oil
- 1 medium onion, finely chopped
- A handful parsley, chopped
- 1 teaspoon turmeric powder
- 3 cups vegetable stock
- Juice, lemon
- 1 eggplant, chopped into chunks
- 1 clove garlic, crushed
- 1 teaspoon smoked paprika
- 7 ounces paella rice
- 1 package chargrilled artichoke
- Lemon wedges to serve

Directions:

1. Place a nonstick pan or paella pan over medium heat. Add 1 tablespoon oil. When the oil is heated, add eggplant and cook until brown all over.

2. Remove with a slotted spoon and place on a plate lined with paper towels.
3. Add 1 tablespoon oil. When the oil is heated, add onion and sauté until translucent.
4. Stir in garlic and parsley stalks. Cook for 10 minutes. Add all the spices and rice and stir-fry for a few minutes until rice is well coated with the oil.
5. Add salt and mix well. Pour half the broth and cook until dry. Stir occasionally.
6. Add eggplant and artichokes and stir. Pour remaining stock and cook until rice is tender. Add parsley leaves and lemon juice and stir.
7. Serve hot with lemon wedges.

Nutrition: Calories 431 Fats 16 g Carbohydrates 58 g Proteins 8

Dessert Recipes – Phase 2

Apple-Raisin Cake

Preparation time: 15 minutes

Cooking time: 50 minutes

Servings: 12

Ingredients:

- One teaspoon baking soda
- 1/2 cups applesauce (no sugar added)
- Two small Golden Delicious apples, cored, pared, and shredded
- 1 cup less 2 tablespoons raisins
- 2/4 cups self-rising flour
- 1 teaspoon ground cinnamon
- 1/2 teaspoon ground cloves 1/3 cup plus 2 teaspoons unsalted margarine
- 1/4 cup granulated sugar

Directions:

1. Spray an 8 x 8 x 2-inch baking pan with nonstick cooking spray and set aside. Into a medium bowl sift together flour, cinnamon, and cloves; set aside.
2. Preheat oven to 350°F. In a medium mixing bowl, using an electric mixer, cream margarine, add sugar and stir to combine. Stir baking soda into applesauce, then add to margarine mixture and stir to combine; add sifted ingredients and, using an electric mixer on medium speed, beat until thoroughly combined. Fold in apples and raisins; pour batter into the sprayed pan and bake for 45 to 50 minutes (until cake is browned and a cake tester or toothpick, inserted in center, comes out dry). Remove cake from pan and cool on wire rack.
3. This cake may be frozen for future use; to make serving easier, slice cake into individual portions, then wrap each portion in plastic freezer wrap and freeze. When ready to use, thaw the number of portions needed at room temperature.

Nutrition: Per serving 151 calories 2 g protein 4 g fat; 28 g carbohydrate 96 mg sodium; 0 mg cholesterol

Apple-Nut Squares

Preparation time:

Cooking time:

Servings: 8

Ingredients:

- 3/4 cup all-purpose flour
- 1 teaspoon double-acting baking powder
- 1 egg
- 2 tablespoons plus
- 2 teaspoons firmly packed dark brown sugar
- 1/2 cup chunky-style peanut butter
- 1 teaspoon vanilla extract
- 1/2 teaspoon ground cinnamon
- 1/4 cup skim milk
- 2 small Golden Delicious apples, cored, pared, and diced

Directions:

1. Preheat oven to 350°F. Onto sheet of wax paper or a paper plate sift together flour and baking powder; set aside.
2. In a medium mixing bowl, combine egg and sugar and, using an electric mixer, beat until thick; add peanut butter, vanilla, and cinnamon and beat until combined. Add sifted

flour alternately with milk, about ⅓ at a time, beating after each addition; stir in apple.

3. Spray an 8 x 8 x 2-Inch baking pan with nonstick cooking spray; spread batter evenly in pan and bake until top is lightly browned, 30 to 35 minutes. Remove pan to wire rack and let cool for 5 minutes; remove the cake from pan and return to rack to cool completely. Cut into sixteen 2-inch squares.

Nutrition: 184 calories 7 g protein 9 g fat 21 g carbohydrate

Yogurt-Fruit Pie

Preparation time: 15 minutes

Cooking time: 6 minutes

Servings: 8

Ingredients:

Crust

- 16 graham crackers, made into crumbs
- 1/2 cup thawed frozen concentrated orange juice (no sugar added)
- 2 tablespoons plus 2 teaspoons granulated sugar
- 1 envelope unflavored gelatin

Topping

- 40 small seedless green grapes
- 2 small nectarines, pitted and sliced
- 2 tablespoons plus 2 teaspoons margarine, softened
- 2 cups plain low-fat yogurt
- 1/2 cup canned crushed pineapple (no sugar added)
- 1 teaspoon vanilla extract
- 1/4 cup sliced strawberries

Directions:

1. To Prepare Crust: Preheat oven to 350°F. Spray 9-inch glass pie plate with nonstick cooking spray; set aside.
2. In small bowl combine crumbs and margarine, mixing thoroughly; using the back of a spoon, press crumb mixture over bottom and up sides of sprayed pie plate. Bake until crust is crisp and brown, about 10 minutes; remove to wire rack and let cool.
3. To Prepare Filling: Pour orange juice into a small saucepan. Combine sugar and gelatin and sprinkle over juice; let stand for 1 minute to soften. Cook over medium-low heat, constantly stirring, until sugar and gelatin are completely dissolved; set aside.
4. In a medium bowl, using a wire whisk, gently stir together yogurt and pineapple; add gelatin mixture and vanilla and stir until thoroughly blended. Pour mixture into cooled pie crust; cover and refrigerate until firm, overnight or at least 4 hours.
5. To Serve: Arrange fruit decoratively over filling; serve immediately or cover and refrigerate until ready to use.

Nutrition: Per serving 202 calories 6 g protein 6 g fat 33 g carbohydrate

Potato Rosettes

Preparation time: 15 minutes

Cooking time: 0 minutes

Servings: 4

Ingredients:

- 8 ounces sliced pared potatoes, cooked and drained
- 2 tablespoons buttermilk
- 1 tablespoon plus 1 teaspoon each grated Parmesan cheese, divided, and margarine
- 1/2 teaspoons each minced fresh parsley and frozen or chopped fresh chives
- 1/4 teaspoon salt
- Dash white pepper

Directions:

1. Force potatoes through a food mill or coarse sieve into a 1-quart mixing bowl; add milk, 1 tablespoon cheese, and the margarine and seasonings and combine thoroughly.
2. Spray baking sheet with nonstick cooking spray.-Fit a pastry bag with a large rosette tube and fill the bag with potato mixture; pipe out mixture onto the sheet, forming 8 spiral cones, each about 2 inches In diameter (if pastry bag is not available, spoon potato mixture onto the sprayed sheet, forming 8 mounds). Sprinkle each potato cone (or mound with 1/2 teaspoon cheese and broil, about 6 inches from the heat source, just until golden brown.

Nutrition: Per serving 88 calories 2 g protein 4 g fat

Creamy Peanut Dip

Preparation time: 15 minutes

Cooking time: 0 minutes

Servings: 4

Ingredients:

- 1 tablespoon lemon juice
- 1/2 cup plain low-fat yogurt
- Dash vanilla extract
- 1/4 cup smooth peanut butter
- 3 tablespoons water
- 2 tablespoons thawed frozen concentrated orange juice (no sugar added)

Directions:

1. In a small bowl, combine peanut butter, water, and juices, mixing until smooth, stir in yogurt and vanilla. Cover and refrigerate until chilled.
2. Delicious served with fresh fruit (e.g., apples, pears, bananas, etc.) or carrot and celery sticks.

Nutrition: Per serving 126 calories 6 g protein 8 g fat

Stuffed Dates

Preparation time: 15 minutes

Cooking time: 0 minutes

Servings: 4

Ingredients:

- 8 pitted dates, split open lengthwise
- 1/2 teaspoon confectioners' sugar
- 1/4 cup smooth peanut butter
- 2 teaspoons grated fresh orange peel, divided

Directions:

1. In a small bowl, combine peanut butter and 1 teaspoon orange peel; spoon 1/2 of the mixture into each date. Sift an equal amount of sugar over each filled date, then sprinkle each with 1/2 of the remaining orange peel.

Nutrition: Per serving 141 calories 5 g protein 8 g fat 16 g carbohydrate

Other Recipes – Phase 1

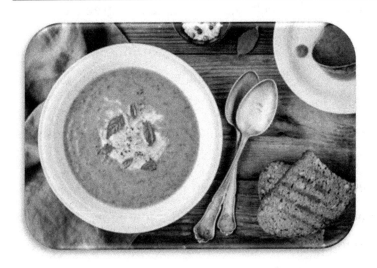

Soup 'Green

Preparation Time: 15 minutes

Cooking time: 0 minutes

Servings: 1

Ingredients:

- Water in sufficient quantity to achieve the desired texture
- 1 green apple with skin
- 1 slice of fresh peeled ginger
- Half lemon or 1 lime without skin, the white part without seeds
- Half cucumber with skin

- Half bowl of leaves with fresh spinach
- 1 bunch of basil or fresh cilantro
- 1 branch of wireless celery, including tender green leaves

Directions:

1. Wash and chop all the ingredients. Insert them into the glass of blender and crush.
2. Add the water and crush again until you get a homogeneous texture. If necessary, rectify water.
3. Take the soup as a snack at any time of the day to purify the body and keep cravings at bay. To know more: This cold soup is quick to prepare and has great benefits for the body. Perhaps the best-known property of the apple is its intestinal regulatory action. If we eat it raw and with skin, it is useful to treat constipation, since this way we take advantage of its richness in insoluble fiber present in the skin, which stimulates the intestinal activity and helps to keep the intestinal muscles in shape. Also, green apples are one of the largest sources of flavonoids. These antioxidant compounds can stop the action of free radicals on the cells of the body. Eating raw fruits and vegetables is the healthiest option.

Nutrition: Calories 330 Fat 12 g 18 % Cholesterol 90 mg Sodium 240 mg 10 % Carbohydrate 20 g 6 % Fiber 5 g 22 % Sugars 4 g Iron 15 %

Pea Salad, Gourmet Peas, Grapefruit

Preparation time: 20 minutes

Cooking time: 10 Min

Servings: 6

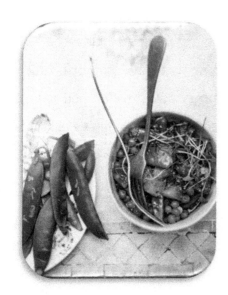

Ingredients:

- 1 pink grapefruit
- 800 g shelled peas
- 200 g gourmet peas
- 2 fresh onions with the stem
- 1 tray of sprouted seeds
- 1 drizzles of olive oil
- 1 dash of apple cider vinegar
- 1 tablespoon old-fashioned mustard

- Seeds sesame toasted

Directions:

1. Peel the grapefruit and collect the flesh (without the white skin), as well as the juice.
2. Steam peas 3-4 minutes and gourmet peas a little more
3. Mix the mustard in a salad bowl with the grapefruit juice, olive oil, vinegar, salt and pepper. Add the chopped onions with the stem, the vegetables and the grapefruit flesh. Mix well, sprinkle with sesame and sprinkle with sprouted seeds.

Nutrition: Calories: 1 Cal / Pers.

Detoxifying Milkshake

Preparation time: 10 minutes

Cooking time: 0 minutes

Servings: 2

Ingredients:

- 1 cup of Celery (one head)
- 2 glass of Spinach
- 2 glass of Cucumber
- 1 unit (s) of Limón
- 2 unit (s) of Apple
- 1 pinch of fresh ginger

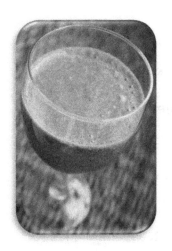

Directions:

1. Put the ingredients – Celery, Spinach, Cucumber, Limón, Apple, fresh ginger in the blender and then blend till a homogeneous mixture is obtained.

Nutrition: Composition Amount (gr) CDR (%) Calories 191.21 10% Carbohydrates 29.52 9.5% Proteins 7.32 15.3%

Green Pineapple Smoothie

Preparation time: 5 minutes

Cooking time: 0 minutes

Servings: 1

Ingredients:

- 50 grams of Chard
- 1 unit (s) of Apple
- 200 grams of Pineapple
- 1 teaspoon of Flax seeds

Directions:

1. Add Chard, Apple, Pineapple, Flax seeds all to the glass of the blender with a little water and grind well.

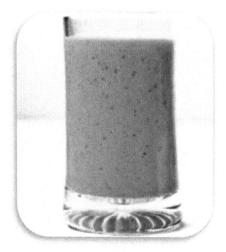

Nutrition: Calories 251.16 13.1% Carbohydrates 46.44 14.9% Proteins 3.51 7.3%

Other Recipes – Phase 1

Cream of Pear and Arugula

Preparation Time: 20 minutes

Cooking time: 0 minutes

Servings: 2

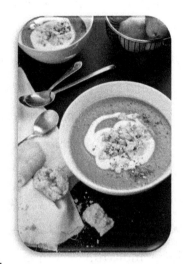

Ingredients:

- Half a liter of water
- 1 bowl of arugula
- The juice of 1 small lemon
- Sea salt or herbal salt
- 1 pinch of ground black pepper
- Extra virgin olive oil
- Edible flowers to decorate
- 4 pears Banuelos with leather, at its point of maturation
- 2 tablespoons of fresh aromatic herbs

Directions:

1. Grind whole the ingredients in the blender jar, except extra virgin olive oil and flowers, until a creamy and homogeneous texture is obtained. If necessary, rectify water, salt, and pepper.
2. Refrigerate until ready to serve and, once in the bowl, decorate with the flowers and a thread of olive oil. If you do

not have flowers, you can use chopped almonds, some rocket leaves or sesame seeds.

3. If you do not have a bowl of arugula you can also use other green leaves such as spinach, lamb's lettuce, watercress, mustard greens, etc. with the aromatic herbs, the same: you can make with parsley, dill, chives, basil, cilantro or mint. To know more: The pear is a fruit with satiating effect for its fiber content: it is fantastic for people who want to lose weight and are doing a diet to lose weight. Also, it is a fruit with anti-inflammatory action, helps us maintain a regular intestinal transit and combat constipation, and has a very beneficial effect on our micro biota or intestinal flora. Choose it whenever you can from organic farming.

Nutrition: Calories197.1 Total Fat12.1 g Saturated Fat3.2 g Polyunsaturated Fat3.5 g Monounsaturated Fat4.1 g Cholesterol10.0 mg Sodium181.2 mg Potassium149.7 mg Total Carbohydrate21.3 g Dietary Fiber3.0 g Sugars15.9 g Protein3.5 g

Chocolate Cupcakes with Matcha Icing-Sirt Food

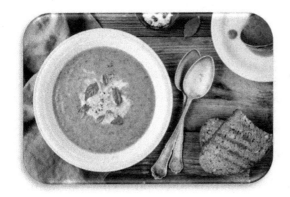

Preparation time: 10 minutes

Cooking time: 20 minutes

Servings: 12

Ingredients:

- 150g self-rising flour
- 200g wheel sugar
- 60g cacao
- 1/2 tsp. salt
- 1/2 tsp. excellent espresso coffee, decaf if chosen
- 120ml milk
- 1/2 tsp. vanilla extract
- 50ml grease.
- One egg
- 120ml boiling water
- For the topping:
- 50g butter, at room temperature level.
- 50g topping sugar
- 1 tbsp. Matcha eco-friendly tea powder
- 1/2 tsp. vanilla bean paste

- 50g soft cream cheese

Directions:

1. Preheat the stove to 180C/160C follower.
2. Place the flour, sugar, chocolate, salt and also espresso powder in a big bowl and mix thoroughly.
3. Include the milk, vanilla extract, vegetable oil and egg to the dry active ingredients and use an electric mixer to defeat until well-integrated. Very carefully pour in the boiling water slowly as well as beat on a low rate until completely incorporated. Make use of broadband to defeat for a more minute to include air to the batter. The batter is a lot more liquid than a regular cake mix. Have faith; it will certainly taste fantastic!
4. Spoon the batter uniformly in between the cake cases. Each cake instance ought to be no more than 3/4 full. Bake in the stove for 15-18 minutes, till the combination gets better when tapped. Remove from the oven and also enable to cool down entirely before icing.
5. To make the topping, lotion the butter and topping sugar together until it's pale and also smooth. Add the Matcha powder as well as vanilla and stir once again. Finally, add the lotion cheese as well as defeat up until smooth. Pipeline or topped the cakes.

Nutrition: 234 Cal

Other Recipes – Phase 1

Other Recipes – Phase 1 (Part 2)

Creamy Strawberry & Cherry Smoothie

Preparation time: 10 minutes

Cooking time: 15 minutes

Servings: 1

Ingredients:

- 100g 3½ oz. strawberries
- 75g 3oz frozen pitted cherries
- 1 tablespoon plain full-fat yogurt
- 175mls 6fl oz. unsweetened soya milk

Directions:

1. Place the ingredients into a blender then process until smooth. Serve and enjoy.

Nutrition: 132 calories per serving

Grapefruit & Celery Blast

Preparation time: 10 minutes

Cooking time: 15 minutes

Servings: 1

Ingredients:

- 1 grapefruit, peeled
- 2 stalks of celery
- 50g 2oz kale
- ½ teaspoon Matcha powder

Directions:

1. Place ingredients into a blender with water to cover them and blitz until smooth.

Nutrition: 71 calories per serving

Orange & Celery Crush

Preparation time: 10 minutes

Cooking time: 15 minutes

Servings: 1

Ingredients:

- 1 carrot, peeled
- 3 stalks of celery
- 1 orange, peeled
- ½ teaspoon Matcha powder
- Juice of 1 lime

Directions:

1. Place ingredients into a blender with enough water to cover them and blitz until smooth.

Nutrition: 95 calories per serving

Tropical Chocolate Delight

Preparation time: 10 minutes

Cooking time: 15 minutes

Servings: 1

Ingredients:

- 1 mango, peeled & de-stoned
- 75g 3oz fresh pineapple, chopped
- 50g 2oz kale
- 25g 1oz rocket
- 1 tablespoon 100% cocoa powder or cacao nibs
- 150mls 5fl oz. coconut milk

Directions:

1. Place ingredients into a blender and blitz until smooth. You can add a little water if it seems too thick.

Nutrition: 427 calories per serving

Walnut & Spiced Apple Tonic

Preparation time: 10 minutes

Cooking time: 15 minutes

Servings: 1

Ingredients:

- 6 walnuts halves
- 1 apple, cored
- 1 banana
- ½ teaspoon Matcha powder
- ½ teaspoon cinnamon
- Pinch of ground nutmeg

Directions:

1. Place ingredients into a blender and add sufficient water to cover them, blitz until smooth and creamy.

Nutrition: 95 calories per serving

Coq Au Vin

Preparation time: 10 minutes

Cooking time: 15 minutes

Servings: 8

Ingredients:

- 450g 1lb button mushrooms
- 100g 3½oz streaky bacon, chopped
- 16 chicken thighs, skin removed
- 3 cloves of garlic, crushed
- 3 tablespoons fresh parsley, chopped
- 3 carrots, chopped
- 2 red onions, chopped
- 2 tablespoons plain flour
- 2 tablespoons olive oil
- 750mls 1¼ pints red wine
- 1 bouquet grain

Directions:

1. In a large plate, put the flour and coat the chicken in it. Heat the olive oil then add the chicken and brown it, before setting aside. Fry the bacon in the pan then add the onion and cook for 5 minutes. Pour in the red wine and add the chicken, carrots, bouquet grain and garlic. Transfer it to a large ovenproof dish. Cook at 180C/360F for an hour. Remove the bouquet grain and skim off any excess fat, if necessary. Add in the mushrooms and cook for 15 minutes. Stir in the parsley just before serving.

Nutrition: 459 calories per serving

Turkey Satay Skewers

Preparation time: 10 minutes

Cooking time: 15 minutes

Servings: 2

Ingredients:

- 250g 9oz turkey breast, cubed
- 25g 1oz smooth peanut butter
- 1 clove of garlic, crushed
- ½ small bird's eye chili or more if you like it hotter, finely chopped
- ½ teaspoon ground turmeric
- 200mls 7fl oz. coconut milk
- 2 teaspoons soy sauce

Directions:

1. Combine the coconut milk, peanut butter, turmeric, soy sauce, garlic and chili. Add the turkey pieces to the bowl and stir them until they are completely coated. Push the turkey onto metal skewers. Place the satay skewers on a barbeque or under a hot grill broiler and cook for 4-5 minutes on each side, until they are completely cooked.

Nutrition: 431 calories per serving

Salmon & Capers

Preparation time: 10 minutes

Cooking time: 15 minutes

Servings: 4

Ingredients:

- 75g 3oz Greek yogurt
- 4 salmon fillets, skin removed
- 4 teaspoons Dijon Mustard
- 1 tablespoon capers, chopped
- 2 teaspoons fresh parsley
- Zest of 1 lemon

Directions:

1. Put the yogurt, mustard, lemon zest, parsley and capers in a mixing bowl. Thoroughly coat the salmon in the mixture. Place the salmon under a hot grill broiler and cook for 3-4 minutes on each side, or until the fish is cooked. Serve with mashed potatoes and vegetables or a large green leafy salad.

Nutrition: 321 calories per serving

Moroccan Chicken Casserole

Preparation time: 10 minutes

Cooking time: 15 minutes

Servings: 4

Ingredients:

- 250g 9oz tinned chickpeas garbanzo beans drained
- 4 chicken breasts, cubed
- 4 Medrol dates, halved
- 6 dried apricots, halved
- 1 red onion, sliced
- 1 carrot, chopped
- 1 teaspoon ground cumin
- 1 teaspoon ground cinnamon
- 1 teaspoon ground turmeric
- 1 bird's-eye chili, chopped
- 600mls 1 pint's chicken stock broth
- 25g 1oz corn flour
- 60mls 2fl oz. water
- 2 tablespoons fresh coriander

Directions:

1. Place the chicken, chickpeas garbanzo beans, onion, carrot, chili, cumin, turmeric, cinnamon and stock broth into a large saucepan. Put it to the boil, and reduce heat after that simmer for 25 minutes. Add in the dates and apricots and simmer for 10 minutes. In a cup, mix the corn flour together with the water until it becomes a smooth paste. Pour the mixture into the saucepan and stir until it thickens. Add in the coriander cilantro and mix well. Serve with buckwheat or couscous.

Nutrition: 401 calories per serving

Chili Con Carne

Preparation time: 10 minutes

Cooking time: 15 minutes

Servings: 4

Ingredients:

- 450g 1lb lean minced beef
- 400g 14oz chopped tomatoes
- 200g 7oz red kidney beans
- 2 tablespoons tomato purée
- 2 cloves of garlic, crushed
- 2 red onions, chopped
- 2 bird's-eye chilies, finely chopped
- 1 red pepper bell pepper, chopped
- 1 stick of celery, finely chopped
- 1 tablespoon cumin
- 1 tablespoon turmeric
- 1 tablespoon cocoa powder
- 400mls 14 FL oz. beef stock broth
- 175mls 6fl oz. red wine
- 1 tablespoon olive oil

Directions:

1. Put the oil in a saucepan then add the onion and cook for 5 minutes. Add in the garlic, celery, chili, turmeric, and cumin and cook for 2 minutes before adding then meat then cook for another 5 minutes. Pour in the stock broth, red wine, tomatoes, tomato purée, red pepper bell pepper, kidney beans and cocoa powder. Let it simmer for 45 minutes, keep it covered and stirring occasionally. Serve with brown rice or buckwheat.

Nutrition: 390 calories per serving

Prawn & Coconut Curry

Preparation time: 10 minutes

Cooking time: 15 minutes

Servings: 4

Ingredients:

- 400g 14oz tinned chopped tomatoes
- 400g 14oz large prawns' shrimps, shelled and raw
- 25g 1oz fresh coriander cilantro chopped
- 3 red onions, finely chopped
- 3 cloves of garlic, crushed
- 2 bird's eye chilies
- ½ teaspoon ground coriander cilantro
- ½ teaspoon turmeric
- 400mls 14fl oz. coconut milk
- 1 tablespoons olive oil
- Juice of 1 lime

Directions:

1. Place the onions, garlic, tomatoes, chilies, lime juice, turmeric, ground coriander, chilies and half of the fresh coriander cilantro into a blender and blitz until you have a smooth curry paste. In a frying pan, put the oil, add the paste and cook for 2 minutes. Stir in the coconut milk and warm it thoroughly. Add the prawn's shrimps to the paste and cook them until they have turned pink and are completely cooked. Stir in the fresh coriander cilantro. Serve with rice.

Nutrition: 322 calories per serving

Choc Nut Truffles

Preparation time: 10 minutes

Cooking time: 15 minutes

Servings: 1

Ingredients:

- 150g 5oz desiccated shredded coconut
- 50g 2oz walnuts, chopped
- 25g 1oz hazelnuts, chopped
- 4 Medrol dates
- 2 tablespoons 100% cocoa powder or cacao nibs
- 1 tablespoon coconut oil

Directions:

1. Place ingredients into a blender and process until smooth and creamy. Using a teaspoon, scoop the mixture into bite-size pieces then roll it into balls. Place them into small paper cases, cover them and chill for 1 hour before serving.

Nutrition: 236 calories per serving

No-Bake Strawberry Flapjacks

Preparation time: 10 minutes

Cooking time: 15 minutes

Servings: 1

Ingredients:

- 75g 3oz porridge oats
- 125g 4oz dates
- 50g 2oz strawberries
- 50g 2oz peanuts unsalted
- 50g 2oz walnuts
- 1 tablespoon coconut oil
- 2 tablespoons 100% cocoa powder or cacao nibs

Directions:

1. Place ingredients into a blender and process until they become a soft consistency. Spread the mixture onto a baking sheet or small flat tin. Press the mixture down and smooth it out. Cut it into 8 pieces, ready to serve. You can add an extra sprinkling of cocoa powder to garnish if you wish.

Nutrition: 182 calories each

Chocolate Balls

Preparation time: 10 minutes

Cooking time: 15 minutes

Servings: 1

Ingredients:

- 50g 2oz peanut butter or almond butter
- 25g 1oz cocoa powder
- 25g 1oz desiccated shredded coconut
- 1 tablespoon honey
- 1 tablespoon cocoa powder for coating

Directions:

1. Mix all ingredients into a bowl. Scoop out a little of the mixture and shape it into a ball. Roll the ball in a little cocoa powder and set aside. Repeat for the remaining mixture. Can be eaten straight away or stored in the fridge.

Nutrition: 115 calories per serving

Two-Week Meal Plan – Phase 1 and Phase 2

Let's get to the heart and see a typical food pattern for the whole week. For each day, you will find indicated how much green juice to take and how to organize the main meals indicatively.

As always, it is just an example to adapt according to your tastes and your caloric and nutritional needs.

Phase 1

Day 1-3

- calorie intake is restricted to 1,000 calories.
- Three green juices per day plus one meal.

Day 1: Monday

green juice: 3 cups a day

- **Breakfast:** water + tea or espresso + a cup of green juice;
- **Lunch:** Green juice
- **Snack:** a square of dark chocolate;
- **Dinner:** Moroccan Chicken Casserole + vegetables and chicken.
- **After dinner:** a square of dark chocolate.

Day 2: Tuesday

green juice: 3 times a day

- **Breakfast:** water + tea or espresso + a cup of green juice
- **Lunch:** 2 green juices before dinner;
- **Snack:** a square of dark chocolate;
- **Dinner:** Sirtfood Bites + Coq Au Vin.
- **After Dinner:** a square of dark chocolate.

Day 3: Wednesday

green juice: 3 times a day

- **Breakfast:** water + tea or espresso + a cup of green juice
  Lunch: 2 green juices before dinner;
- **Snack:** a square of dark chocolate;
- **Dinner:** Salmon and Capers + chicken or fish;
- **After dinner:** a square of dark chocolate.

Day 4–7

- Calorie intake is increased to 1,500
- Two green juices per day and two more sirtfood-rich meals

Day 4: Thursday

green juice: 2 times a day

- **Breakfast:** water + tea or espresso + a cup of green juice
- **Lunch:** Sirt Muesli;
- **Snack:** a green juice before dinner;
- **Dinner:** vegetable soup with beans.

Day 5: Friday

green juice: 2 times a day

- **Breakfast:** water + tea or espresso + a cup of green juice

- **Lunch:** buckwheat salad with vegetables;
- **Snack:** a green juice before dinner;
- **Dinner:** grilled fish or meat + a side dish of vegetables and baked potatoes.

Day 6: Saturday

green juice: 2 times a day

- **Breakfast:** a bowl of that delicious Sirt Muesli + a cup of green juice
- **Lunch:** Sirtfood omelette with bacon;
- **Snack:** a cup of green juice;
- **dinner:** chicken with walnuts and parsley + a red onion + tomato salad.

Day 7: Sunday

green juice: 2 times a day

- **Breakfast:** water + tea or espresso + a cup of green juice;
- **Lunch:** Sirt salad + grilled fish or chicken;
- **Snack:** a cup of green juice;
- **Dinner:** fish or meat cooked with a drizzle of red wine + plenty of salad and vegetables.

Phase 2

- You should continue to steadily lose weight.
- No specific calorie limit for this phase.

- You can eat three meals full of sirtfoods and one green juice per day.

Day 8 and 15

- 1 x Sirtfood green juice
- 3 x main meals
- 1 to 2 light bites or appetizers and snacks
- 1 x glass red wine

Smoothie: Creamy Strawberry & Cherry Smoothie

Meal 1: Green Omelet

Meal 2: Courgette Risotto

Meal 3: Roast Balsamic Vegetables

Light Bites: Yogurt-Fruit Pie

Appetizers & Snacks: Apple-Raisin Cake

Day 9 and 16

- 1 x Sirtfood green juice
- 3 x main meals
- 1 to 2 light bites or appetizers and snacks

Smoothie: Mango, Celery & Ginger Smoothie

Meal 1: Sirtfood Breakfast Scramble

Meal 2: Sirtfood Salmon Salad

Meal 3: Chicken Chili

Light Bites: Buckwheat Stir Fry with Kale, Peppers & Artichokes

Appetizers & Snacks: Avocado Deviled Eggs

Day 10 and 17

- 1 x Sirtfood green juice
- 3 x main meals
- 1 to 2 light bites or appetizers and snacks
- 1 x glass red wine

Smoothie: Pineapple & Cucumber Smoothie

Meal 1: Thai Red Curry

Meal 2: Chicken & Bean Casserole

Meal 3: Artichoke & Eggplant Rice

Light Bites: Apple-Nut Squares

Appetizers & Snacks: Creamy Peanut Dip

Day 11 and 18

- 1 x Sirtfood green juice
- 3 x main meals
- 1 to 2 light bites or appetizers and snacks
- 1 to 2 squares dark chocolate (85% cocoa)

Smoothie: Strawberry & Citrus Blend

Meal 1: Sirtfood Omelette

Meal 2: Chia, Quinoa & Avocado Salad

Meal 3: Foil Baked Salmon

Light Bites: Walnut and Onion Tartine

Appetizers & Snacks: Broccoli Cheddar Bites

Day 12 and 19

- 1 x Sirtfood green juice
- 3 x main meals
- 1 to 2 light bites or appetizers and snacks
- 1 x glass red wine

Smoothie: Mango, Celery & Ginger Smoothie

Meal 1: Honey Chili Squash

Meal 2: Brown Basmati Rice Pilaf

Meal 3: Mussels in Red Wine Sauce

Light Bites: Potato Rosettes

Appetizers & Snacks: Stuffed Dates

Day 13 and 20

- 1 x Sirtfood green juice
- 3 x main meals
- 1 to 2 light bites or appetizers and snacks
- 1 to 2 squares dark chocolate (85% cocoa)

Smoothie: Orange & Celery Crush

Meal 1: Cranberry & Orange Granola

Meal 2: Arugula, Egg, and Charred Asparagus Salad

Meal 3: Fried Sardines with Olives

Light Bites: Herb-Roasted Olives and Tomatoes

Desserts: Frozen Strawberry Yogurt

Day 14 and 21

- 1 x Sirtfood green juice
- 3 x main meals
- 1 to 2 light bites or appetizers and snacks
- 1 x glass red wine

Smoothie: Summer Berry Smoothie

Meal 1: Granola - The Sirt Way

Meal 2: Chilli Con Carne

Meal 3: Salmon and Capers

Light Bites: Walnut & Spiced Apple Tonic

Appetizers & Snacks: Tropical Chocolate Delight

Conclusion

Thank you for making it to the end. A healthy meal contains a lot of vegetables. So, most of the plate should consist of vegetables such as zucchini, cucumber, peppers or other vegetables, this guarantees a lot of vitamins, low calories, and a nice freshness (if the vegetables are not overcooked).

Colorful. Of course, it is not enough just to eat vegetables; it should also be varied and colorful. Ideally, the vegetables are as mixed and colorful as a traffic light: yellow, red, and green. Of course, a white vegetable such as white cabbage and cauliflower is not wrong and also serves as a colorful icing on the cake. The colorful mixture, which changes over and over again, also offers many vitamins and a varied taste. Even if you love something (such as tomatoes), it's important to vary a bit. Otherwise, deficiency symptoms can occur, and the food becomes boring over time.

Protein. Protein is one of the essential components of our body. However, not as much as needed, as many believe. And even then, it does not always have to be animal protein.

Other sources of protein from beans and tofu provide a change in the daily diet and bring creativity to life.

Carbohydrates. Again, and again, the diets with "low-carb" (pronounced the "little-carbohydrates") the total hit. No wonder.

Carbohydrates also make you fat. At least if you eat too many of them, if you eat them in the wrong combination (i.e., with too much fat or sugar) or do not vary enough. Carbohydrates are generally crucial in order for us to have energy, an essential ingredient for satiety, and it's important because it's good for your nerves, among other things. Of course

The best thing you can do for your body is to win food from natural ingredients. Fruits and vegetables are, at best, varieties that are available regionally and seasonally. Of course, it is okay from time to time sometimes not to eat regional specialties, such as pineapple or bananas (if you live in Germany, there will probably be hardly regional) but it is completely superfluous outside the strawberry time overpriced strawberries from Africa to buy, which taste like nothing and have hardly any vitamins.

As we end this book, please remember the five no-goes:

A lot of fat

Fat is good for the body. If we have too little fat, it will harm our health in the long run. But many people have the problem of eating too much fat which is not healthy either. Obesity is a modern disease that can easily turn into obesity. Too much fat is bad for the brain, the immune system, and the arteries, which in turn can cause a heart attack.

Of course, one must distinguish between healthy fats (olive oil, nut oil, nuts) and unhealthy fats (butter, animal fats, etc.). Because fat is not the same fat.

Lots of sugar

It is perfectly okay to consume sugar. Because sugar is an energy supplier, and sugar tastes good too. However, too much sugar is not good for the body, the immune system and can lead to addiction in particularly bad cases. Above all, sugar has the disadvantage that it does not fill you up for long and that you quickly lose energy again. Even if you are pushed by sugar, the effect lasts only very briefly.

Chemical substances

Our body is a natural organism; it does not need any chemical additives, so why should you forcefully pump yourself with chemistry? Unfortunately, for convenience, many people tend to stuff themselves with ready-made sauce-fix bags and other unhealthy things. From time to time, it may not be a problem to feed a little unhealthy; you will not die because you incorporate some e-substance. However, too many chemical foods are not good for your health. This can cause many other diseases of affluence that you would not normally have.

Many spices

People like spicy food, and that's perfectly fine, but certain levels of spiciness and too much salt are not among the spices people need on the contrary. The man needs a little salt. In fact, pretty much all foods contain some salt naturally and the over-flavoring of food causes water retention, is bad for the brain, and has a negative effect on the organism.

One-sided

The worst you can do to yourself, and your body is to eat one-sidedly. It does not matter whether the food bathes in fat, whether you are constantly fed on peppers, eating too much sugar or too little fruit, any form of one-sided diet has the result that you have deficiency symptoms, and you get sick sooner or later becomes. This can be in a one-sided diet, where you eat only unhealthy things and in a one-sided diet in which you eat only healthy food. Because one-sided is and remains one-sided. That cannot and should not be the goal because ironing out these deficiencies requires a lot of work and a lot of discipline.

That's all and I hope you have learned something!

CPSIA information can be obtained
at www.ICGtesting.com
Printed in the USA
LVHW050249291120
672741LV00006B/330